D0291864

THE BEVERLY HILLS EXERCISE BOOK

THE
BEVERLY

HILLS EXERCISE BOOK

By ROBERTA KRECH
with Bill Libby

THE BOBBS-MERRILL COMPANY, INC.
Indianapolis / New York

Library of Congress Cataloging in Publication Data

Krech, Roberta.
  The Beverly Hills exercise book.

  1.Exercise. 2.Physical fitness.
I.Libby, Bill. II.Title.
GV481.K73   613.7'1   81 – 17977
ISBN 0 – 672 – 52709 – X   AACR2

DESIGNED BY BERNARD SCHLEIFER
PHOTOGRAPHS BY WEN ROBERTS, PHOTOGRAPHY, INC.

First printing

Manufactured in the United States of America

ACKNOWLEDGMENTS

The authors wish to thank Roberta's husband, John, who helped in many ways. They wish to thank Ernie and Lyn Caron for their help. They wish to thank Wen Roberts of Photography, Inc., who took all the photos. And they wish to thank Bill Adler, who put the idea together.

*For my father and mother, who gave me love
and confidence;*

*For my husband and children, who gave me
encouragement and support;*

*For all those I have met along the way who had a positive
attitude toward life and who have helped me to
pursue my goals with a positive attitude.*

R.K.

CONTENTS

CONTENTS

PART TWO: PARTS OF THE BODY

PART THREE: SOMETHING SPECIAL

THE
BEVERLY
HILLS
EXERCISE
BOOK

INTRODUCTION

BEVERLY HILLS is a very special community located southwest of Hollywood, south of the Santa Monica Mountains, and north of the Pacific Ocean. Much of it consists of hills and valleys and narrow, winding streets, all of which helps to make it exclusive. The brightest stars of the entertainment and business worlds live here. Accordingly, the community boasts world-famous stores and dining spots.

Beverly Hills symbolizes success. The glamorous folk who call it home live in the finest houses, drive the finest cars, wear the finest clothes, and eat the finest food. They want the best, whether it be in things, experiences, or beauty — and they can afford it.

Yet the Beautiful People of Beverly Hills are not by nature better than the rest of us. Nor are they that different really. For the most part, they have attained their positions either because they were lucky, or because they were goal-oriented. They either fell into the good life, or they worked for it. Most of them reached for it — they stretched for success.

With the help of this book you too can reach for the youthful look, the slender, supple figure, the balanced beauty that characterizes the fashionable women who came to my Christine Valmy Salon on Wilshire Boulevard in the heart of Beverly Hills. And, frankly, it will cost you a whole lot less.

My own stretch for success began at the age of seventeen when I was a senior in high school. One day as I was getting off the school bus, a boy said to me, "Bobbie, you're built like a pear!"

That made me angry. But as I seethed over his remark, I realized that just as I was entering the most important period of my life, when I should have been at my best, I had let my body get into terrible shape.

At that moment I decided to change. I went on a diet to lose the thirty extra pounds I had been carrying around. I started to study physical fitness and took exercise and dance classes. At Ohio State University where I went after graduating from high school, I studied physical therapy. At the university I met John Krech, my future husband, whose interests were similar to my own. Together we learned about physical conditioning and nutrition, and subsequently we opened beauty and figure salons throughout the Midwest and East.

After studying for a time under the brilliant Christine Valmy in New York, my husband and I launched the first Christine Valmy Salon in Southern California, in Beverly Hills, right across the street from the famed I. Magnin.

Our salon provided luxurious beauty treatments, and I feel every aspect of beauty, including good nutrition and weight control, skin care and cosmetics, is vital. However, since I firmly believe that exercise is the most essential element in good health and a good appearance, I have chosen to make it the basis for this book. And because exercise creates good skin tone as well as good muscle tone, I have included a chapter on skin care at the end of the book.

Actually, there is little new to offer in the way of exercise, and many exercise books have been published. What I hope will make this one better and more useful to you than many of the others is that I have carefully fit together specific exercises that are most convenient to do at different times of day in whatever physical situations you find yourself. They are a balanced series, designed to correct particular problems. None are difficult to do. When exercises are presented as having degrees of difficulty, it makes them sound important. The fact is, the simplest and most natural exercises work best for your body.

Nearly all of the exercises I have chosen are stretching exercises: some will lengthen your muscles and strengthen your joints to make you loose and limber, and others will trim you down and tone you up. I have little interest in power exercises that build muscle. Those are mostly for men.

Finally, I present the exercises so that you can do a few at this time, a few at that time; some at home and some at the office. Doing them several times during the day — sometimes even while you are engaged in other activities — all adds up to a good day's worth of fitness without your having had to find an hour or two for a massive, monotonous workout.

The beautiful people who came to our Beverly Hills salon wanted to present an attractive appearance to the world, and I made it possible. They were, in the main, busy women who led full lives, who wanted to learn how to fit the most beneficial of beauty regimens into their active days. They may or may not have had more money than you but there is no need for them to have had exclusive access to the secrets of a fine figure and beautiful look. I want to provide you with those same secrets, whether you live in Beverly Hills or Boise, Southern California or Florida, San Francisco or New York, or cities in between.

INTRODUCTION

Most of my prominent clients trust me to protect their privacy, but just to name a few. One was Pam Dawber, the pert, trim Mindy of television's "Mork and Mindy." (The first time one of my young children saw her in person, she asked, "What is she doing out of the box?") Another client was Pia Zandora, a blockbuster Las Vegas singer and entertainer whose vigorous exercise routines keep her in top form. Also, beautiful actress and top model Christina Ferrer. And Marcy Niarchos, an athletic lady from one of the wealthiest families in the world.

Among those I choose not to identify were actresses, singers, and dancers; working women who have positions of power in some of the most important entertainment and business corporations in the country; and the wives of some of the wealthiest, most important and powerful men in the world. Perhaps you fit into one of these groups; perhaps not. But whatever your life-style, you share with them the desire to look and feel your best.

You will have to set high goals for yourself and then reach high to attain them. I will make it as easy for you as I possibly can. But you will have to help.

I am reminded of the Rice brothers of Houston, two-foot-tall midgets with a superb sense of humor. One day they walked into a tall-man's clothing store in Texas and began looking around. When a startled clerk asked if he could help them in any way, they said simply, "No, we're just setting our goals."

Whatever your physical problem, be it a small bust or large tummy, be as positive as the Rice brothers. You *can* set realistic goals, whether it is building up your bust or slimming down your derrière, and you can attain them by following the simple exercises I present for you.

I have been where you are. I am no longer built like a pear, but I do not have the finest figure in the world, nor the most beautiful face. However, I felt comfortable posing for the photographs in this book. I am thirty-two and have given birth to three daughters. I weighed 120

18

pounds before each of their births and weighed the same soon again afterward. I am 5 feet, 8 inches tall, and my measurements have been 36 – 25 – 35 for many years now.

Our figures get tested by life now and then, but we can pass these tests. I partake of the good life, and I am sorely tempted to stray from the straight and narrow at times, as we all are. So I have to keep working continually to stay in shape, because I want to look as good as I can in business suit or swimsuit, jeans or shorts, evening gown or nightgown.

I am healthy and I feel wonderful. I have all the energy I need to lead an active, varied life to the fullest. In fact, in my thirties I feel better than I did at twenty. I believe that when I am forty I can feel as I did at thirty. So can you as you pass the milestones of your life.

You will not have to work hard, but you will have to work consistently. People who come to me and jump into a flurry of furious exercising soon wear themselves down and drop out. Invariably, those who start slowly and gradually develop their routines stick to them and get the most benefit.

You might wish to ask the advice of your physician, particularly if you have any specific problems with your health, before beginning to exercise. But most people are encouraged to begin a good exercise program and stay with it. In the following chapters, I give you one you will enjoy, one you will want to integrate into your schedule permanently.

TIMES
OF DAY

1
EARLY MORNING

BEGIN YOUR NEW DAY right. Ease into it. Riches of one kind or another may lie ahead of you, but don't rush into things. If you have to set an alarm, set it to give you a few extra minutes.

Horizontal Stretch

Start with a stretch, a HORIZONTAL STRETCH. Sit up, yawn, and stretch like a cat, slowly. Stretch from the tips of your fingers to your toes. Stretching is the most natural sort of exercise. It lengthens muscles which have contracted during your night's sleep. Yawning fills your lungs with air. It also exercises your facial muscles. Breathe deeply; it invigorates you by increasing your body's supply of oxygen. As you stretch, point your fingers and reach for the ceiling. (Figure 1.) Inhale deeply as you reach up. Hold each stretch for several seconds. Exhale as you relax. If you have a bed partner, stretch with your partner. Be generous; share exercise.

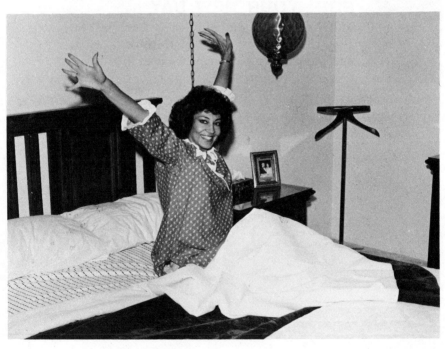

Figure 1.

Alternate Leg Raises

Now lie down and do some ALTERNATE LEG RAISES. These are not as strenuous as conventional leg raises, but they will stretch your leg muscles, strengthen your joints, and slim your thighs and waist. Do not put your hands behind your head as you ordinarily would. Instead, let your arms lie loosely at your sides. Raise one leg vertically overhead, pointing your toes to the ceiling. (Figure 2.) Concentrate on stretching the leg to its fullest extension. (As with each of this series of exercises, inhale through the nose as you move up, and exhale through the mouth as you move down. Deep breathing is fundamental to each exercise.) Hold your leg in the extended position for three counts, lower it slowly, then raise the other leg and repeat the exercise. Begin by doing five lifts for each leg. Gradually increase the number to ten for each leg.

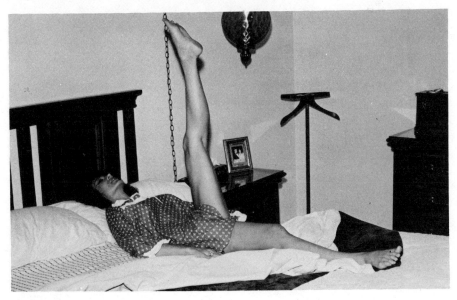

Figure 2.

Alternate Leg Curls

Now do some ALTERNATE LEG CURLS. Still lying flat on your back, arms placed loosely at your sides, bring each leg up in turn, with knee bent and toes pointed. (Figure 3.) Hold this position for a count of five. This loosens your leg muscles and strengthens your thigh and stomach muscles. It is also time to do something for your upper body muscles, and this is a good preliminary exercise to the following one. Both exercises are good for those dimples that form on the sides of your derrière. (Dimples are delightful on the face, but not on the derrière.) Do the Alternate Leg Curl five times for each leg.

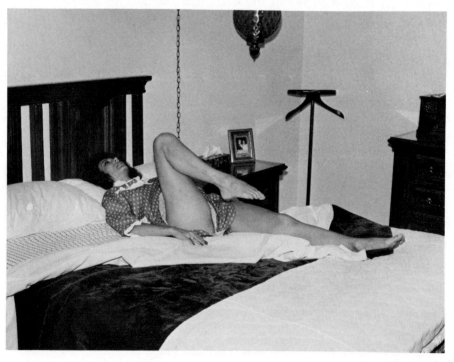

Figure 3.

Arm-Leg Hugs

Next come the ARM-LEG HUGS. Lying on your back, raise one leg with knee bent. Clasp your knee with both hands and press your thigh toward your chest. As you do so, raise your head and draw your forehead toward your knee. (Figure 4.) Hold this position for a count of three. Release and slowly lower your leg. Repeat this exercise with the other leg. Do five Arm-Leg Hugs with each leg and over a period of time build up to ten repetitions for each leg. This is an excellent early-day and all-around exercise. You can feel the stretching in your thighs, arms, shoulders, back, and neck. But do not stretch to extreme tension on this or any other exercise in this book; stretch just enough to feel it.

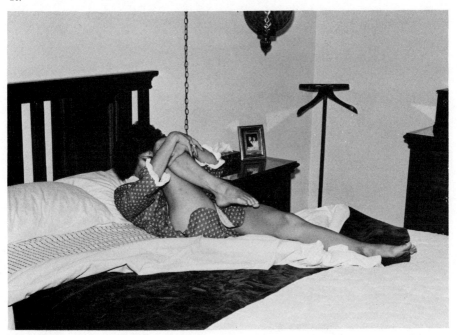

Figure 4.

Sit-Reaches

Finally, before getting out of bed, do a few SIT-REACHES. Sit up and stretch your arms overhead, then lean forward. Reach until your fingertips come as close to your toes as you can manage. (Figure 5.) Hold this position for a count of five. Do not force yourself to reach farther than you can go comfortably, but you should feel some tension along the tops of your thighs and through your arms, your shoulders, your back, even your buttocks. Return slowly to your seated position, arms down. Raise your arms and repeat the exercise for a total of five times. This exercise is effective in reducing your derrière and slimming your waist, as well as stretching and limbering your muscles for the day's activities. You are now ready to get out of bed, your first big move of the day. You should feel loose, relaxed, and ready to go.

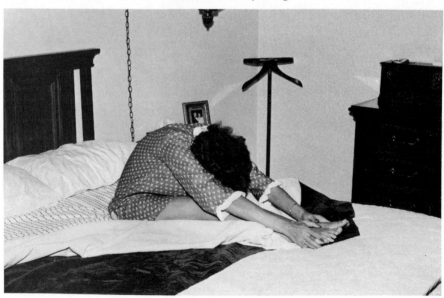

Figure 5.

2

AFTER
RISING

NOW THAT YOU'RE OUT of bed, let's really loosen up and stretch to meet the day. Standing exercises are excellent for limbering up the joints, getting a good supply of oxygen flowing throughout the body, and stimulating blood circulation.

Standing Stretch

Start with a STANDING STRETCH. With legs spread, first stretch your arms straight out to the sides, then up over your head. (Figure 1.) Finally bend forward, letting your arms drop down toward the floor, hands loosely clasped. (Figure 2.) Every muscle in your body is being stretched, but move slowly, without stressing yourself. Stretch just to the point of feeling tension.

Feel your rib cage lift as you reach up with your arms and inhale through your nose. Exhale through your mouth as you drop forward.

Every part of your body is benefiting from this exercise. It is especially good for spinal mobility. Practice it slowly, concentrating on full extension in each stretch. At first do five standing stretches, and in time work up to ten each morning.

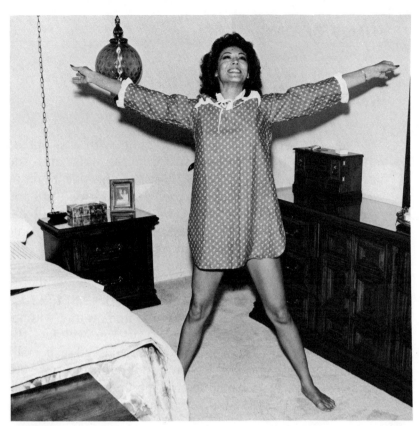

Figure 1.

Figure 2.

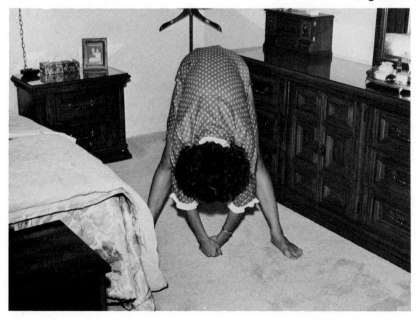

Rotations

Now, ROTATIONS. Standing straight, with legs spread and hands on hips, bend forward from the waist until you are facing the floor. (Figure 3.) Bend to one side as far as you can (Figure 4), and then rotate to the back until you are looking up at the ceiling. Continue to rotate until you are leaning on the opposite side (Figure 5), then come around to the forward position again. Return to the upright position. Imagine that you are drawing a gigantic, continuous circle with the top of your head. Remember to return to the upright position at the end of each full rotation. If you just continue to go around and around without straightening up, you may get dizzy. You will feel the blood moving up to your brain, which isn't bad, especially to start the day. You will loosen and stretch most of your muscles, work your waistline, and loosen your lower back. Do three rotations at first, increasing the number to six.

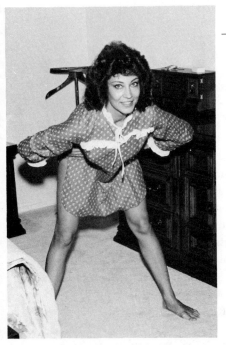

Figure 3.

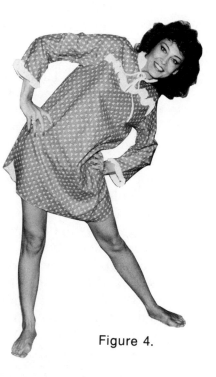

Figure 4.

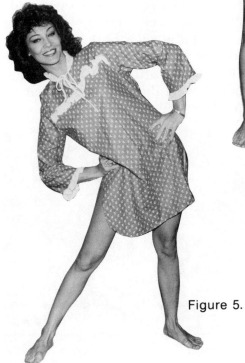

Figure 5.

33

Funny Faces

It's time to shower and dress. A warm shower is a wonderful way to wake up and get a clean, fresh start. Pause before entering the shower to make a few funny faces in the mirror. This is not to amuse yourself as much as it is to exercise facial and neck muscles which are not often used. Certain movements will help to smooth wrinkles and eliminate double chins. We will get into these FUNNY FACES later in Chapter 8, which deals with the face, chin, and neck. But this is a good time to introduce this exercise, because you look into a mirror first in the morning, usually in the bathroom area, and you can make these faces most effectively by doing them in front of a mirror. Clench your teeth and raise your chin as high as you can. Watch the muscles strain as you stretch your underchin and neck muscles. (Figure 6.) Now blow out through nearly closed lips (Figure 7), then yawn wide (Figure 8), and suck in your cheeks (Figure 9), holding each position at full strain for a count of three. Men are not so prone toward double chins as are women, by the way, and one reason is that they stretch their underchin and neck muscles while shaving their faces. For good results, women can copy those stretching movements.

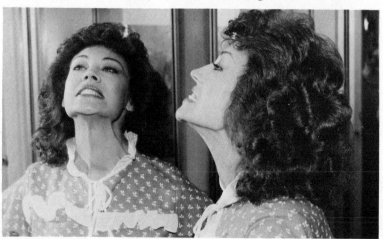

34

Figure 6.

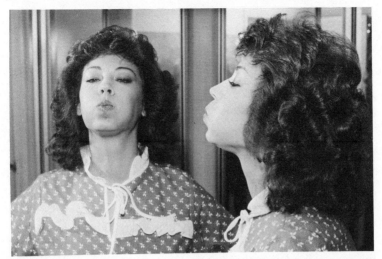

Figure 7.

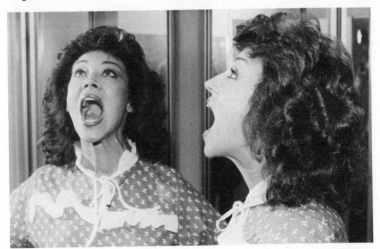

Figure 8.

Figure 9.

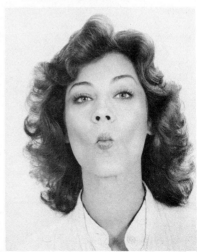

Arm Scissors

Fresh from your shower, you may have to dress now for work or for other activities. But if you have the time, here are two more exercises that will ease you into the day. They may also be done prior to your shower, while you are still in your nightgown or pajamas, of course. The first is the ARM SCISSORS. It is good for general loosening up, as well as for trimming the sides of your waistline and for removing the flabby tissue that forms on the backs of your upper arms. Standing with your legs comfortably apart, balance on the balls of your feet and lift your arms up with hands stretched outward. (Figure 10.) Bring your heels down to the floor, at the same time lowering your arms and crossing them in front of you. (Figure 11.) Again, rise up on your toes, swinging your arms up to the outstretched position, then return to the arms-crossed position once more. Do five complete scissors, increasing eventually to ten repetitions.

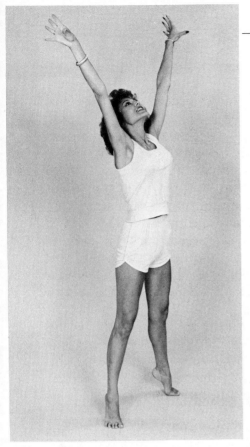

Figure 10.

Figure 11.

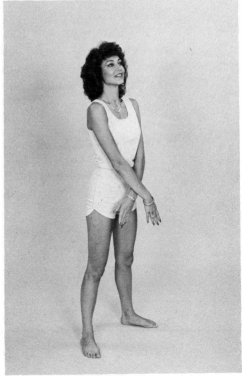

Reclining Leg Scissors

The last exercise is the RECLINING LEG SCISSORS. Lying on your back with hands flat at your sides, raise your legs, spread them wide (Figure 12), and scissor them all the way across each other. (Figure 13.) Open them wide again, and scissors them across, repeating this movement five times before returning your legs to the floor. While doing this exercise, spread your legs until you feel the tension in your thighs, then cross them until you feel the tension in your buttocks. This is good for the thighs and buttocks. Eventually increase the number of scissor movements to ten at a time.

Other exercises good to do at this time might be the Seated Leg Extensions of Chapter 3, the Seated Horizontal Scissors Kick and Leg Extensions of Chapter 5, the Leg Extensions of Chapter 9, the Shoulder Shrugs and Rib Cage Raises of Chapter 11, and the Side Bends of Chapter 16.

By now you will have warmed up, stretched, and awakened your lower body as well as your upper body, your legs as well as your arms. You're on your way to health, wealth, and happiness.

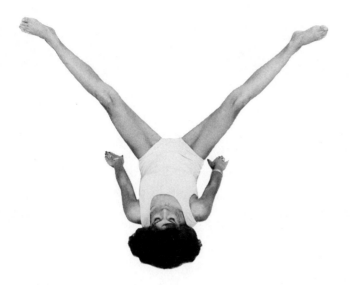

Figure 12.

Figure 13.

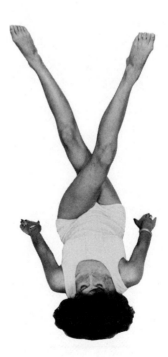

3
WORKDAY, MIDDAY

MOST DAYS ARE WORKDAYS eight to ten hours long for many of us, whether we live in Beverly Hills or Baltimore. Much of the day is spent standing or sitting in one position. I'm a bit more active than the average person, because I have conducted private physical conditioning classes for clients for many years. However, many people, whether they are executives or secretaries, may be busy all day long without being physically active; or their physical activity may be the kind that does not condition them. One woman film studio executive told me, "I run around so much that by the end of the day I can't walk a block." If these people would steal five minutes here and five minutes there during the workday to exercise, they would find themselves refreshed, able to work better with energy left over at the end of the workday. If you're in this position, steal the time. Let's call it a cosmetic crime!

41

Head Presses

HEAD PRESSES can be done at a desk at work, while waiting in a car at a traffic light, or while watching television. You may not want to do them when anyone is watching, but be sure to take a minute's time for this excellent tension reliever. Simply place the palm of one hand against the side of your head and press up with the palm while pushing down with your head. (Figure 1.) Now, repeat this movement on the other side. Next, place your hand on your forehead and apply pressure. Then, place your hand on the back of your head and press. Finally, repeat all the positions using both hands (Figure 2) to apply pressure. You will be surprised how much better you feel for it. Your entire upper body — shoulders, neck, hands, arms, and head — is involved. Apply steady pressure for five seconds in each position. Relax for five seconds. Resume. Strike each position once or twice.

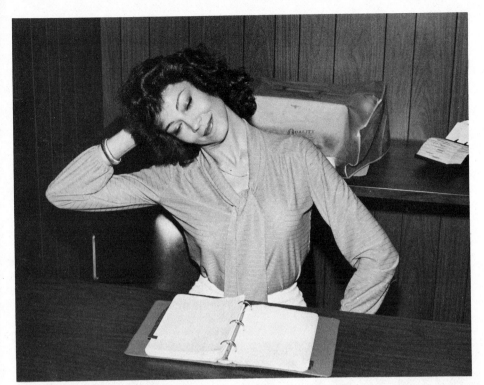

Figure 1.

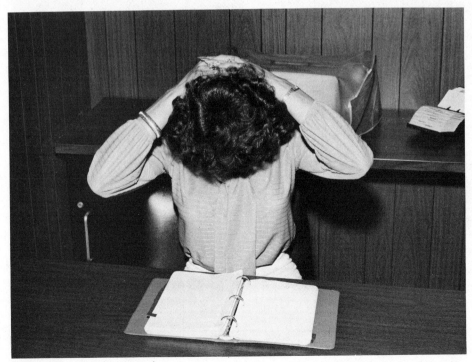

Figure 2.

Head Stretches

Similarly, HEAD STRETCHES will relieve tension and relax you. With your hands on your hips, gently roll your head back (Figure 3) and hold the position for five counts. Then, gently drop your head forward and hold for five more counts. Repeat each movement five times. Sound simple? Perhaps too simple? Simplicity is the secret to the success of many exercises. This one works; many of the more complex exercises do not. This one may be new to you. Don't do it when anyone might be watching. You'll look as though you'd fallen asleep on the job!

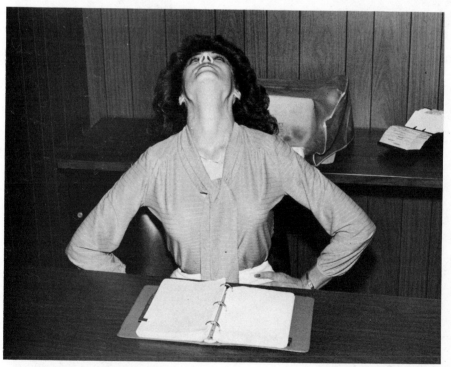

Figure 3.

Seated Leg Extensions

A bit more vigorous are SEATED LEG EXTENSIONS. These are very helpful for the waist, abdomen, and thigh muscles. Sit in a straight-back, armless chair. Firmly grasp the chair seat on either side. Keeping your back straight, lift your knees slightly (Figure 4), then

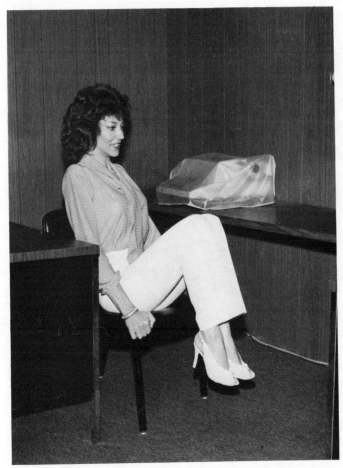

Figure 4.

45

straighten your legs so that they are extended at a slight upward angle. (Figure 5.) Hold for a count of three, then slowly lower your legs. Concentrate on achieving a full extension of your legs. You will feel stress through your buttocks, too. The tension you feel in your muscles will help to arrest that dread disease, secretary's spread. As with the other exercises, inhale in the upward motion and exhale in the downward movement. Start with three seated Leg Extensions and increase to six.

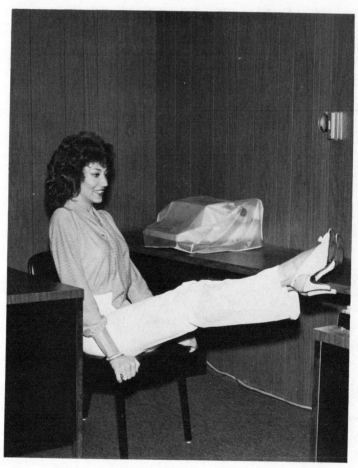

Figure 5.

Side Leg Extensions

When no one is around, try some simple standing exercises. Stand with one hand on a chair for balance and the other on your hip. (Figure 6.) Raise the leg you are

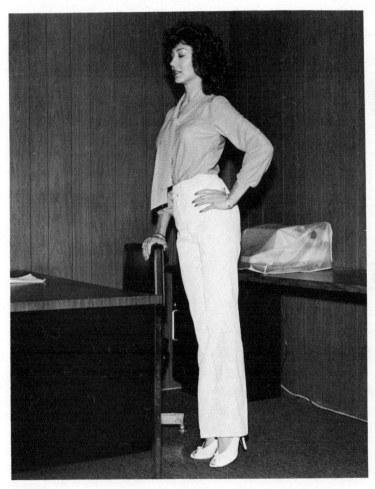

Figure 6.

resting your hand on out to the side (Figure 7), hold for a count of two, then bring it down. Do ten to one side, then switch and do ten to the other side. Do these in rapid, rhythmic succession. Concentrate on stretching each leg out as far as possible — out, not up. Side Leg Extensions can also be done while filing, cooking, washing dishes. They will help to reduce the so-called saddle-bags that form around the hips and thighs.

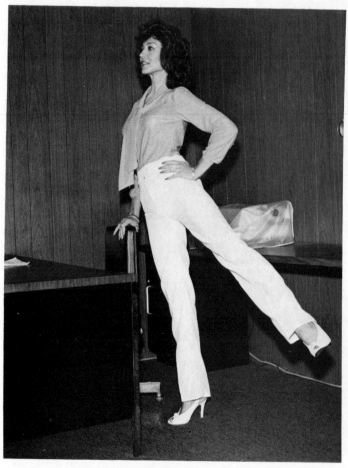

Figure 7.

Back Leg Extensions

Now for BACK LEG EXTENSIONS. Grasping a chair, extend one leg directly behind you. (Figure 8.) Stand as straight as possible, and keep your extended leg as straight as possible. Hold for a count of two. Bring the leg down and repeat the extension with the other leg. Do five repetitions with each leg and eventually increase to ten. Do the extensions briskly, yet concentrate on extending your leg fully, with knee straight and toes pointed. These too can be done at a counter, while cooking or washing dishes, while waiting at the copying machine, while doing a dozen things that do not benefit your body one bit but which do have to be done. Consider these exercises as things that have to be done, too.

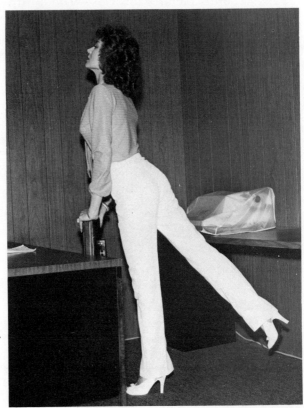

Figure 8.

Partial Pushups

If you're really gung-ho, go for some PARTIAL PUSHUPS. Stand with your palms flat at the edge of a desk and your legs behind you at a 45-degree angle. (Figure 9.) Start with arms straight and gradually bend them until you have lowered your abdomen to the edge of the desk. (Figure 10.) Without leaning against the desk, hold the position for a count of three, then push yourself back up with your arms. Do five pushups at first and build up to ten. Keep your back straight. Inhale as you come up, exhale as you go down. Do these slowly for greatest effect. This exercise is good for the arms, shoulders, bust, ankles and feet.

Also, as long as you're going this far, you might try some facial exercises — the Funny Faces described in Chapters 2 and 8. This could, of course, set you apart from your co-workers. And scare away some customers. But if *you* don't do something for your face, who will?

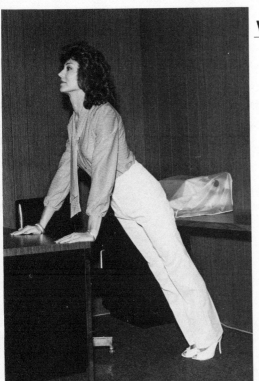

Figure 9.

Figure 10.

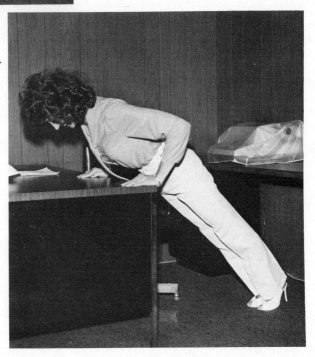

4
ON THE WAY

N SOUTHERN CALIFORNIA, bus and train transportation leave a lot to be desired, so we spend a lot of time in our cars — going to work and back, flitting here and there. To a certain extent, this traveling time is wasted.

Of course, it is not wasted if you can cruise the backcountry of the hill people off Sunset Boulevard or drive along Benedict Canyon Road, where you will glimpse some truly majestic mansions. But the traffic along the main thoroughfares of Wilshire Boulevard, Sunset Boulevard, and Santa Monica Boulevard is bumper-to-bumper. And since Beverly Hills would not permit itself to be spoiled by freeways, you have quite a distance to travel to reach the San Diego, Ventura, and Hollywood freeways which take you to other parts of Southern California.

There are some people who refuse to waste the time they spend in the car, though. Jack Kent Cooke, who now and in the past has owned professional football, baseball, basketball, and hockey teams and sports arenas, lived in

Beverly Hills before moving to Washington, D.C. He always employed a chauffer so that he could conduct business by telephone while on the road. Many producers, directors, and other executives of the film industry in Hollywood do likewise. One actress who comes to the Christine Valmy Salon tapes her lines and plays them back on a cassette player in her car so that she can memorize them while driving. Other Southern Californians catch up on the latest Rona Jaffe novel or learn to speak Spanish while stuck in traffic jams.

Why not exercise? Obviously, there are exercises that cannot be done with any degree of safety while driving a car. But there are some that you can do, especially while stopped at red lights or tied up in the kind of traffic jams that confront drivers every day in Beverly Hills or on the freeways.

Steering Wheel Push

These exercises involve the upper body, especially the arms, shoulders, neck, head, and face. First try the STEERING WHEEL PUSH. With your hands gripping the upper portion of the steering wheel, push straight back until you feel the tension in your arms, shoulders, and neck. (Figure 1.) This movement also strengthens the wrists and hands. Hold for a count of five, then relax. Repeat. Now, gently roll your head back until you are facing the ceiling of the car and you can feel the tension in your neck and underchin. (Figure 2.) Hold for a count of five, then relax. Repeat. Be sure you do the exercises only when the car is stopped! Not only will these movements lengthen and strengthen a lot of muscles, but you will find they will relieve a lot of tension.

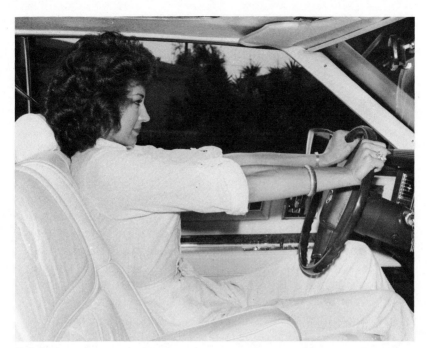

Figure 1.

Figure 2.

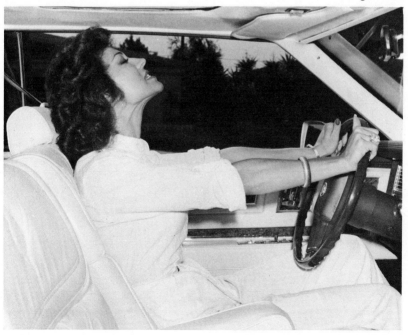

More Steering Wheel Pushes

Another version of the STEERING WHEEL PUSH can be done by inclining the head hard to the left (Figure 3), then to the right, while pressing forcefully on the steering wheel. (Figure 4.) Make the most of each press by pursing your mouth, as in some of those Funny Faces you make to exercise seldom-used jaw and mouth muscles. These Steering Wheel Pushes can be done while driving, too. But you may cause some consternation to others driving nearby. When driving, I sometimes draw unwanted whistles, mouthed comments, or compliments from other drivers. I counter with a few Funny Faces, which scare the heck out of them. One woman in New York takes no chances with suspicious-looking people who approach her. She starts talking loudly to herself and crazily shaking her head. People take the long way around her, including, I suspect, some would-be muggers or purse snatchers.

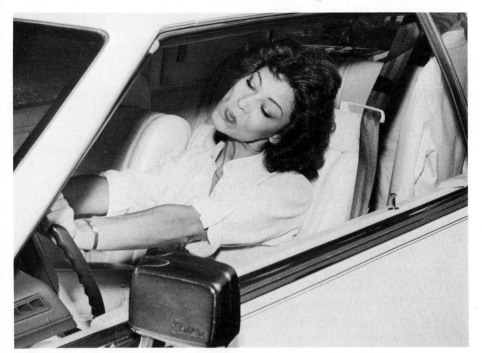

Figure 3.

Figure 4.

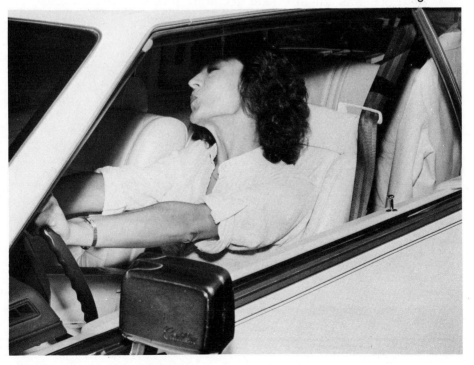

Steering Wheel Pulls

A similar exercise, the STEERING WHEEL PULL, can be done by gripping the bottom half of the steering wheel and pulling, instead of gripping the top half and pushing. This is good for the bust line, as well as the arms and shoulders. You will feel the tension across your chest. You can get added benefit by thrusting your head backward or forward. When your head is thrown back, you will feel the tension in the muscles in the front of your neck and in your face. (Figure 5.) When your head falls forward, you will feel the tension at the back of your neck and through your chin. (Figure 6.) Thus these movements are good for firming up neck muscles and avoiding or reducing a double chin. Of course, you shouldn't do these while the car is in motion, or you will look like I do in Figure 6. If ever there was an after-the-accident picture, this is it! So choose a safe moment for road exercises.

For additional exercises while en route, check out the Funny Faces described in Chapters 2 and 8. Also try the Shoulder Shrugs described in Chapter 11.

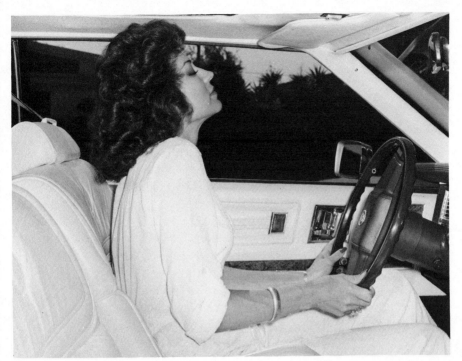

Figure 5.

Figure 6.

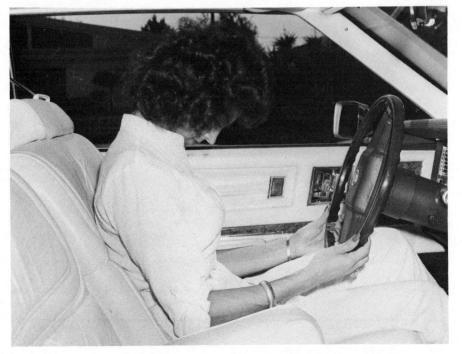

5

EARLY
EVENING

EXERCISES for the late-afternoon or early-evening blahs may be just what you need to get the most out of your evening hours. Whether you work at home or in an office, whether you have been on your feet or sitting all day, here are exercises that will make you feel like dancing — or at the least keep you awake until bedtime. Many of my most glamorous clients had to look their best after dark. Hollywood's round of glittering parties, film premieres, and other social highlights required them to look bright-eyed, fresh, and relaxed. You'll want to be ready to enjoy the evening's activities, too, whether it means a night on the town or an evening at home with family or friends.

Seated Horizontal Scissors Kick

Begin by sinking into your favorite easy chair. Don't just collapse there. Oh, all right, collapse. But just for a minute. Now, let's energize and get the juices boiling. Let's start with a SEATED HORIZONTAL SCISSORS KICK. Sit forward toward the edge of the chair, head up, back straight, hands gripping the arms of the chair. In these photographs I'm sitting back in the chair — I need to rest sometimes! — but you should sit forward in your chair with your back straight. Raise your legs slightly. Cross one leg over the other. (Figure 1.) Then, swing your legs wide apart. (Figure 2.) Cross your legs again, this time with the other leg on top. (Figure 3.) Do ten scissors kicks in a fairly rapid continuous flow. You will feel the strain on your inner thighs and abdomen. You will be tightening your hips, thighs, and abdomen. You will be flattening your tummy. Eventually build the number of scissors kicks to twenty. This is not too strenuous, yet is superb exercise.

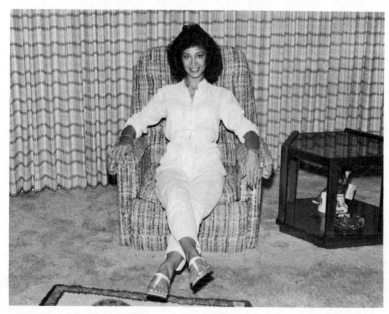

Figure 1.

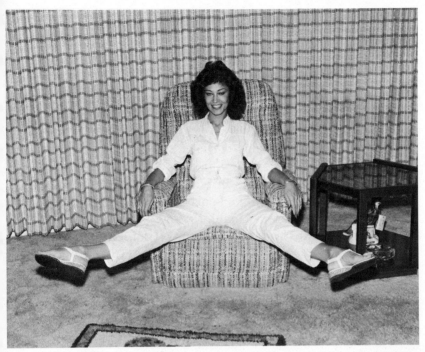

Figure 2.

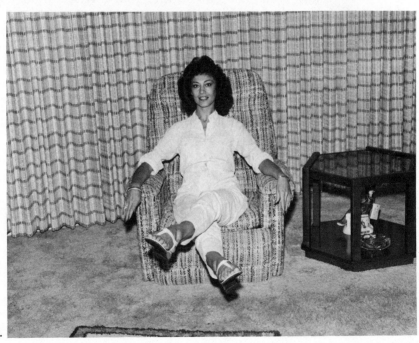

Figure 3.

Seated Leg Extensions

Now, let's try some SEATED LEG EXTENSIONS. Like the previous exercise, not only is this a good late-afternoon or early-evening refresher, but it can be done effectively while watching television, for example, or talking on the telephone, or even reading a book. You should concentrate on each exercise in order to get the most out of it, but you can also make the most of your time by doing some of the exercises while engaged in other activities. Again, seated on the edge of a chair and gripping the arms, raise your legs, bending your knees up to face level and pointing your toes toward the floor. (Figure 4.) Then, extend your legs so that your knees are straight, your feet are at face level, and your toes are pointed toward the ceiling. (Figure 5.) Now, relax and slowly lower your feet to the floor. Repeat the exercise five times, eventually building to ten at a time. Seated Leg Extensions are rather strenuous. Concentrate on raising your legs as high as possible in the first phase, then as high and straight as possible in the second phase. Inhale on the way up; exhale on the way down. You will feel the strain in your leg and abdominal muscles, and even in your shoulder, arm, and neck muscles. This exercise really will reduce your waist and abdomen and thin out and strengthen your thighs and calves.

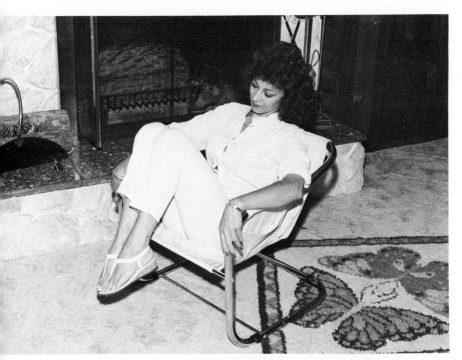

Figure 4.

Figure 5.

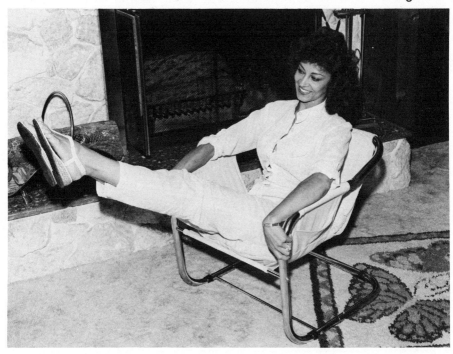

Seated Leg Swings

The next exercise, SEATED LEG SWINGS, is quite easy to do, yet is very invigorating and very good for the waist, hips, and thighs. Sit sideways on one buttock on the edge of a chair, inner leg bent, foot flat on the floor for balance. Swing the outer leg up high and straight, pointing your toes (Figure 6), then swing it back as far as you can, keeping your toes pointed. (Figure 7.) Concentrate on getting full extension in your leg and foot in both directions. Hold each extended position for a count of three. Do five continuous forward and backward extensions. Then turn to face the opposite direction and repeat the exercise with the other leg. Do five leg extensions in each direction, working up to ten in each direction. This exercise is exceptionally good for football punters, ballerinas, and dancers in the chorus line, but it will also do a lot for you.

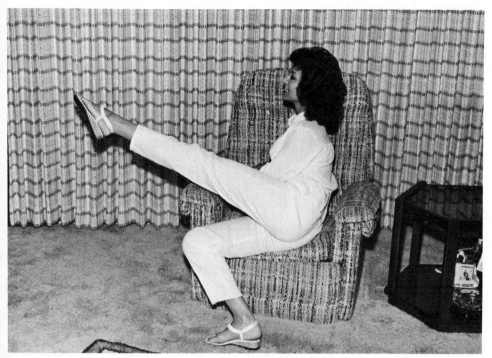

Figure 6.

Figure 7.

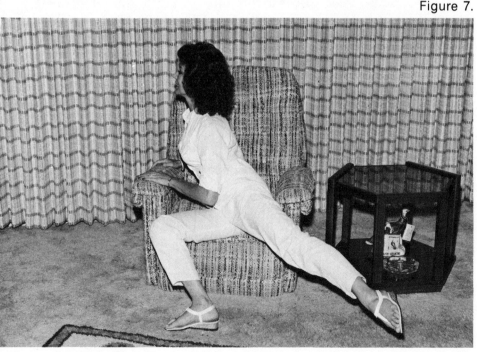

Foot Lifts

Finally, let's do some FOOT LIFTS. These can be effective for relieving tired feet or legs and for lengthening, strengthening, and toning thigh, calf, ankle, and foot muscles. They will also help prevent fallen arches. They can be done at almost any time of the day or night when you feel the need, and they can be done almost any place, including at the filing cabinet, the sink, or when talking on the telephone. Usually, it is helpful to have somewhere to place your fingertips for balance, but you should not press down. Simply rise up on your toes (Figure 8), hold for a count of five, then slowly lower your heels to the floor. Even though you may walk a great deal during the day, you do not use these muscles in just this way. Foot Lifts will help you to stay on your feet longer without becoming tired. Again, this is a great exercise for dancers.

Also good to do at this time would be the Horizontal Stretch of Chapter 1, the Head Presses and Stretches of Chapter 3, the Seated Side and Back Leg Extensions of Chapter 3, the Yoga Sit of Chapter 6, the Cat and Kneeling Stretches of Chapter 7, the Shoulder Shrugs and Rib Cage Raises of Chapter 11, and the Yoga Sits and Hail Heroes of Chapter 17.

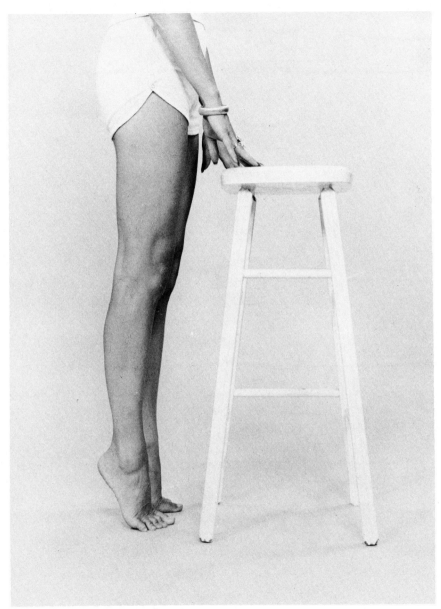

Figure 8.

6

LATE NIGHT

TOO TIRED TO SLEEP? Sometimes at the end of a long day you can't unwind enough to drift off to sleep. Or maybe you are so tense that you can't enjoy a sexual interlude with your partner. Sex is excellent exercise, if you are fortunate enough to have a compatible partner. You can burn up 1,200 to 1,500 calories a session. The more relaxed and limber you are before getting into bed, the better you will be in bed. And the better your shape, the more attractive and appealing you will be. A woman needs curves to accentuate her femininity, but beyond these, the slimmer you are these days, the sexier you are.

Even if it's not a night for romance, or if you're sleeping alone, here are exercises that will relax you and prepare you for a proper night's rest.

Hail Hero

I call the first exercise HAIL HERO. It is a fundamental exercise based on the principles of Yoga. It is superb for the upper torso, the back, and the thighs. Start on your hands and knees (Figure 1), then slowly lower yourself until you are almost sitting on your heels. Bend your head toward the floor and press your chest toward your thighs. Your arms should be extended, palms to the floor. (Figure 2.) Do not sit on your heels. You will feel a lot of pull through your thighs and upper body. The thrust of your body should be forward, not back. Hold this position for a count of ten. Then pull yourself forward until you are up on your hands and knees. Rest for a count of three in that position. Repeat the complete exercise three to five times. Inhale in the raised position just prior to going down; exhale in the lowered position and inhale as you return to your hands and knees.

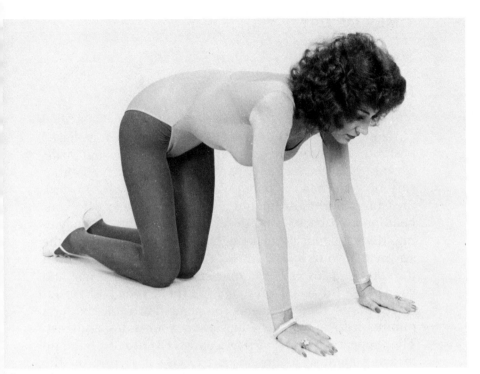

Figure 1.

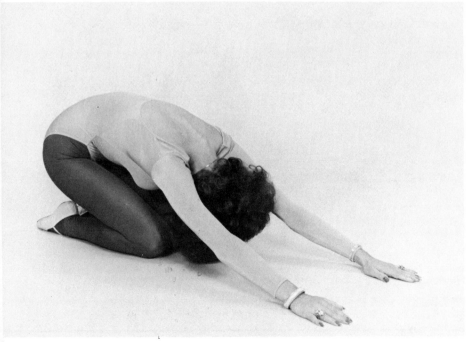

Figure 2.

The Cobra

Now, let's go right into the COBRA, another Yoga-based position. Lie forward on your stomach with your arms close to your body, elbows bent and palms down on either side of your head. Then push yourself slowly upward, thrusting your chest up and arching your back, with your head pressed back. (Figure 3.) Try to look up at the ceiling. Keeping your buttocks tightened will take some of the strain off your lower back. You will feel the stretch through your lower back, your shoulders, your arms, and your neck. Inhale as you come up, hold your position for three counts, then exhale as you come down. Lie flat for a minute with arms down loosely at your sides and rest. Then repeat for a total of four Cobras. Eventually, build up to doing eight at a time. This exercise is terrific for the lower back, bust, and hips and is an excellent relaxer.

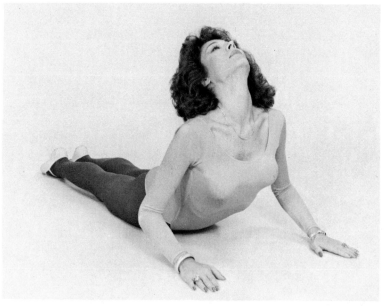

Figure 3.

Yoga Sit

Another relaxer before getting into bed, perhaps the best relaxer of all, is a simple YOGA SIT. This differs from classic Yoga sitting postures in that your arms are up-raised to form a half-circle. Cross your legs in front of you the way old-time tailors did, keeping your back straight. If you can tuck one foot inside the opposite calf, fine. As you lift your arms, lift your upper torso also, raising your rib cage. (Figure 4.) Hold this position for a count of three. Lower your arms until they are crossed in your lap. Relax. This relaxed position is excellent for contemplation, or the "no-thought" that relaxes the mind. There is a point to "contemplating your navel," as they say.

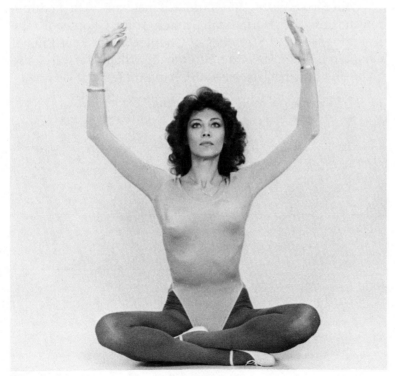

Figure 4.

75

At times when we want to clear our minds, it may be helpful to focus on something that requires little or no thought, such as our navels or a blank wall. Some meditative techniques consist of repeating a mantra, a word or group of words designed to calm the mind and to get the mind and body back into harmony.

At the end of the day, those moments before getting into bed should be relaxing ones. You may want to watch Johnny Carson on television after you get into bed — especially if you have nothing better to do. But I feel a few minutes of soft music to accompany some relaxing exercises or sitting silently in a restful position is beneficial to both mind and body. Many movie and television stars, some of whom come into the Christine Valmy Salon, believe strongly in Yoga. They live under a lot of pressure, and they treasure their relaxation. So should you.

Other exercises that lend themselves to a bedtime routine are the Horizontal Stretch from Chapter 1, the Head Presses and Stretches of Chapter 3, the Foot Lifts of Chapter 5, the Kneeling Stretch of Chapter 7, and the Yoga Sits and Hail Heroes of Chapter 17.

7

AFTER THE BIG NIGHT OUT

WE ALL DO IT; we all overeat or overdrink at times. And in L.A. there are plenty of places to indulge yourself. Ciro's and other famous nightclubs where the stars used to gather to see and be seen are gone, but in their place are many fancy saloons and loud discos where the stylish set can still let its hair down and let it all hang out. No matter where you live, there is a spot or two nearby where you can play into the late hours of the night. And at times we all pay for our overindulgences.

I had a client from a German background who enjoyed spending her evenings in a lively beer parlor where German-style dancing and beer drinking were the custom. She came to me prepared to exercise hard to work off the beer, but she would not give it up. So be it. We can't cut out everything we like and still like our lives. We may have to cut out some things and overcome others. There are exercises you can do that will help you feel better when you have overdone it.

Walking is the best bet. Walking briskly for a reasonable distance will help to digest your food and burn off the alcohol. Beverly Hills is a great place to walk — provided you can find a place to park your car first! And it is still a safe place to walk, even at night, especially along the famous shopping streets of Rodeo Drive, Beverly Drive, Camden Drive, Wilshire Boulevard, and Little Santa Monica Boulevard.

Window shopping at Nieman-Marcus, I. Magnin's or Saks Fifth Avenue; at Gucci's, Georgios, or Battaglia's; at Yves St. Laurent or Yaeger's, or at any of many other fashionable shops — where shoes may go for two hundred dollars and a dress for two thousand — is a wonderful way to work off a few sins. No doubt you have a pleasant street or park somewhere near you.

Rotating Stretches

After walking, you might try some ROTATING STRETCHES to further relieve that stuffed feeling. (One client called it "the failure of a round stomach to adjust to a square meal.") Begin by locking your fingers together so that your palms face outward. Keeping your hands clasped and your knees straight, bend forward from the waist with your arms stretched down toward the floor. Then rotate all the way to one side (Figure 1), straighten up with your arms over your head (Figure 2) and circle from the waist until you are stretching to the other side. (Figure 3.) Rotate slowly as if you were holding a bucket of water in your hands. (In Beverly Hills it might be a bucket of gold, or even oil!) Continue this circular motion until you have made five rounds. This exercise should not be rigorous; if you feel too much tension in the backs of your legs, bend your knees slightly.

Figure 1.

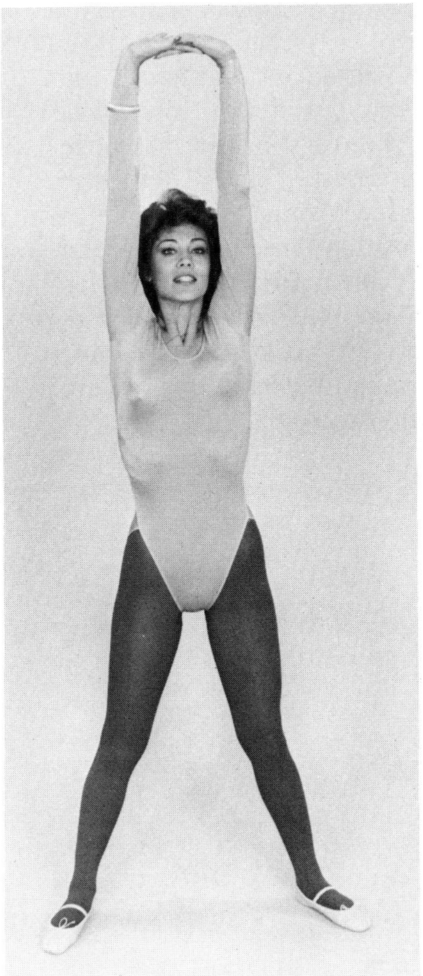

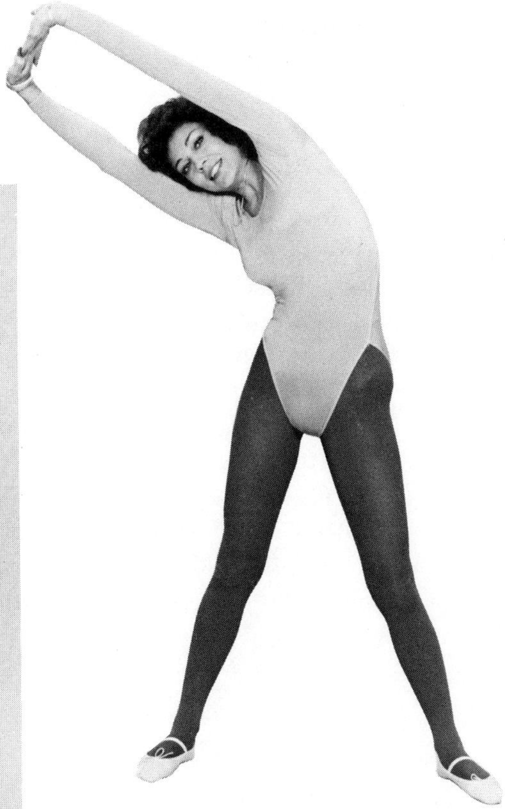

Figure 2.

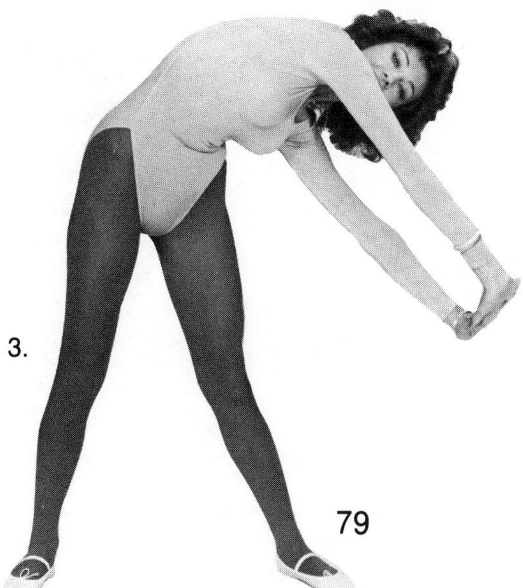

Figure 3.

The Cat

Next, pretend you are a CAT. Kneel on your hands and knees. Raise your back, pressing your chin to your chest and tightening your stomach. (Figure 4.) Don't bother to meeouw, but hold the position for five counts. Return to the relaxed position. Moving slowly, repeat the Cat five times, holding the extended position for five counts each time. Inhale on the way up; exhale on the way down. This is a Yoga posture, and deep breathing is essential. Remember each time to raise your back, tighten your stomach, press down with your chin. By doing this you are raising your rib cage and aiding digestion.

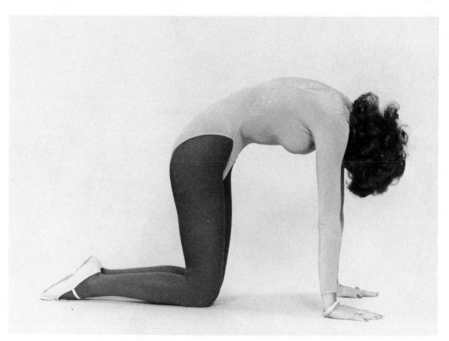

Figure 4.

The Kneeling Stretch

Another good exercise for combating overdrinking and overeating, a condition not exactly rare in affluent Beverly Hills, is the KNEELING STRETCH. Starting on your knees, lean back, raise your hands and thrust them forward. (Figure 5.) Hold this position for a count of three. Bring your hands to your hips as you bring your body upright and relax. Inhale as you move back, exhale as you come forward. Breathe deeply. Fill your lungs with air and your body with oxygen-carrying blood. You're trying to make up for having overloaded yourself. Now you must do what you can to get back into shape as soon as possible. Don't wait around for the feeling to wear off on its own.

Additional exercises you can do to alleviate the effects of overeating and overdrinking are the Standing Stretch of Chapter 2, the Yoga Sit of Chapter 6, and the Rib Cage Raises of Chapter 11.

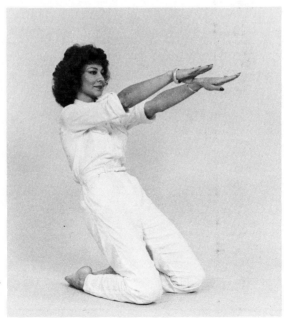

Figure 5.

PART TWO

PARTS OF THE BODY

8

THE FACE, CHIN, AND NECK

WE ARE THE SUM of our parts. None of us measure up to our ideal, not even the glamorous women of the screen who came to my salon. But those women worked to correct their imperfections. One was beginning to get wrinkles on her face; another had started developing a double chin. One had heavy thighs; several had weight problems. Far be it from me to betray their secrets. Or yours. In building beauty we try to maximize our strengths and minimize our weak points. If you're in good shape now, great. It's time to practice preventive medicine. Tone up those facial muscles before they begin to sag, for example. If you have problems, begin working to correct them; or at least try to arrest them before they get worse. It is not a crime to be less than perfect. But it is a crime to be less than you can be, to let yourself go.

PARTS OF THE BODY

Funny Faces

Let's begin with the face. Until recently this was the least exercised part of the body. Now we've begun to realize that the facial muscles are just as much in need of exercise as any other part of the body. We do use many of our facial muscles — when we smile or frown, for example. The problem is we don't use the others. Those we do use create creases — dimples around the mouth from smiling, wrinkles between and around the eyes from frowning, or squinting, or concentrating. The solution is to counteract this tendency by exercising other muscles to achieve a balance between those that are used and those that are not, firming and toning up all the muscles of the face. This can begin in the morning in front of the bathroom mirror with those FUNNY FACES we discussed in Chapter 2, including your best yawn. In Figure 1, I look as though I'm trying to hit high C. It's hard to fake a yawn. But you can try. The yawn not only uses a lot of facial muscles, but also those neglected neck muscles. Strain the neck muscles as you yawn. Hold them in stress for a count of three.

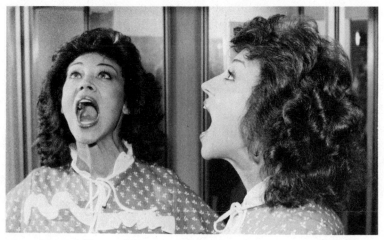

Figure 1.

More Funny Faces

The idea is to make an ugly face in order to have a pretty one. So make more FUNNY FACES — puffing up as though blowing out a candle (Figure 2), then sucking in as though tasting a lemon. There really is nothing funny about these funny faces. They should be taken seriously. They should be done to their extremes, until you feel as much tension as possible in as many facial muscles as possible. Each position should be held to a count of five. Eventually you will discover facial muscles you didn't know you had. If you can locate the couple just in front of the upper part of your ears, you may find you can wiggle your ears. Which will be very helpful if you happen to want to lose weight in your ears.

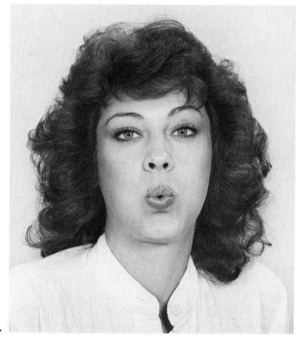

Figure 2.

Neck Twists

Aging often shows up first on the neck and the chin. The muscles below the chin begin to sag into double chins if we tend to be overweight, or into so-called turkey chins if we are not. NECK TWISTS are the best way to firm up these muscles. Pull your head back and your chin up and tense your neck muscles by clenching your teeth. (Figure 3.) Roll your head to one side (Figure 4), back again, then to the other side (Figure 5), maintaining tension all the way. Hold each position for a count of two. Relax. Repeat three times. You will be not only toning these muscles but loosening them, so this is a good early-day exercise.

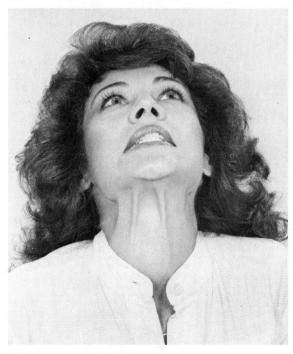

Figure 3.

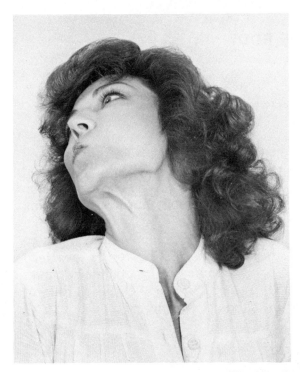

Figure 4.

Figure 5.

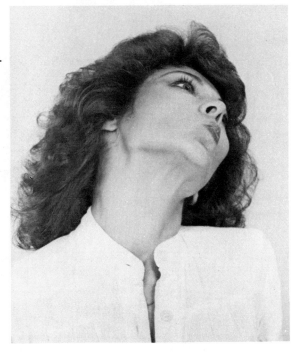

PARTS OF THE BODY

Head Falls

Finally, do some HEAD FALLS. Simply let your head roll to one side (Figure 6), then to the back (Figure 7), and over to the other side. (Figure 8.) Close your eyes. Relax. But don't fall asleep. This is serious business. Wake up, Roberta. Roberta! Wake up!

Additional benefits to the face, chin, and neck can be gained by doing the Rotations of Chapter 2, the Head Presses and Stretches of Chapter 3, the Cobra of Chapter 6, the Shoulder Shrugs of Chapter 11, the Bicycle of Chapter 12, and the Situps of Chapter 17.

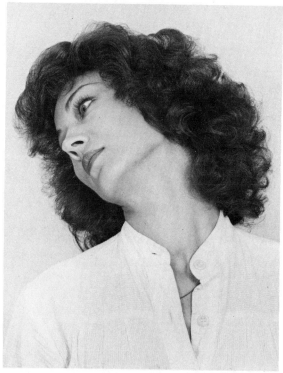

Figure 6.

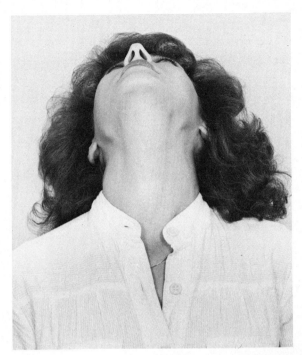

Figure 7.

Figure 8.

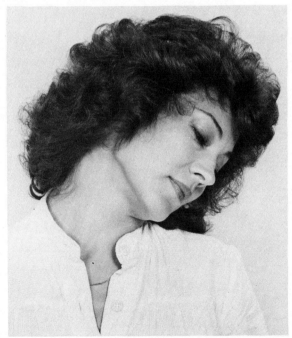

9

THE BACK

STAND UP STRAIGHT! You've heard
this instruction since you were a child, but
you haven't done it. Now is the time to start.
Get into such a habit of standing straight
that you don't have to think about it. Your
posture is the most important aspect of your appearance.
If you slump, every part of you slumps; your breasts and
belly sag. A straight backbone is the foundation of erect
posture. A rounded back and shoulders, in addition to
being unattractive, contribute to back and neck problems.
Those of you who are troubled by backaches and neck-
aches may find relief by strengthening and straightening
your back.

Begin by standing as straight as you can against a flat
wall. Take a posture check. Straighten your head. Pull
your shoulders back and push your chest up, but not too
much; it should feel natural. Place one hand between the
small of your back and the wall. The more room you find
you have to move your hand around, the worse your
posture. If, however, you are carrying a lot of weight in

your derrière, you will not be able to get the small of your back close to the wall. Your problem then is not necessarily poor posture.

The Book Walk

Now, place a book on your head. And walk. (Figure 1.) This is the oldest and best test of good carriage. In order to balance the book as you walk, you will have to be standing up straight, with your head erect, your eyes level. The BOOK WALK will tell you where you stand in developing a straight back and good posture. When you have achieved an erect carriage, you can return to this exercise and execute it easily and effectively — eventually. If you work at it, you can improve your posture considerably.

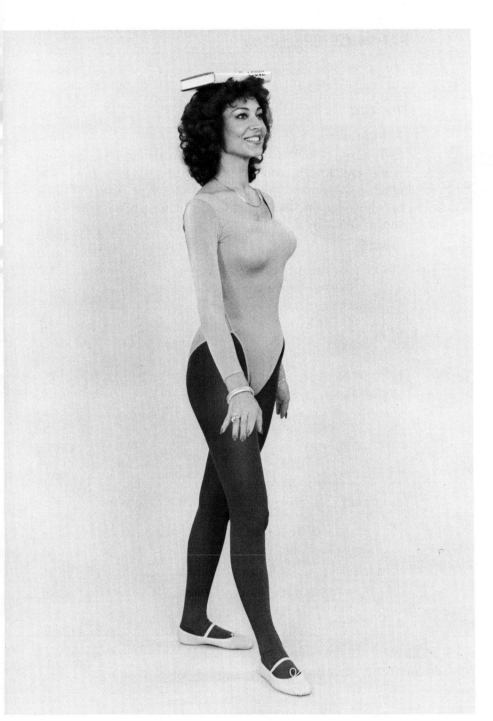

Figure 1.

The Cat

To strengthen your back, begin with the CAT. On your hands and knees, suck in air, raising up your back and holding the tensed position for a count of three. (Figure 2.) Then, let out the air and return to a relaxed posture. Repeat five times.

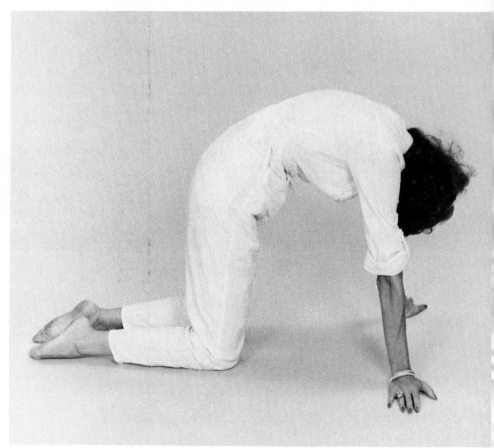

Figure 2.

Back Leg Extensions

Now, do some KNEELING BACK LEG EXTENSIONS. Start on your hands and knees. Bring one knee up to your chest, bringing your head down toward your knee. (Figure 3.) Then thrust your leg straight back and up, pointing your toes and lifting your head high. (Figure 4.) Hold the extension to a count of three, then relax. Do five Back Leg Extensions with each leg.

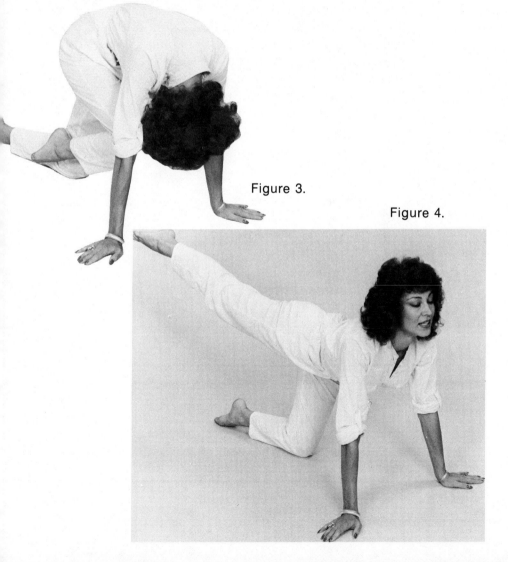

Figure 3.

Figure 4.

PARTS OF THE BODY

Hand Reaches

Drop into a seated position and try some HAND REACHES. Sit with your legs stretched out to the side as far as they will go. Reach with one hand to touch your foot. Then reach with the other hand to touch the other foot. Keep your body centered over your knee and your knee straight. Really stretch, but be careful not to pull a muscle. Now, reach with both hands toward one foot (Figure 5), then toward the other. (Figure 6.) Try to grasp your ankle each time, and hold each position for a count of three. You will feel the stretching in your back, shoulders, arms, and legs. This will give you flexibility through your back and hips and will tighten your back, waist, thighs, and upper arms. Repeat each position five times.

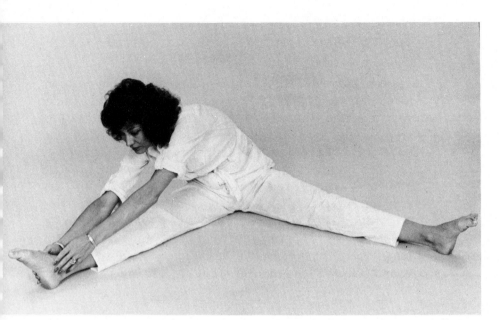

Figure 5.

Figure 6.

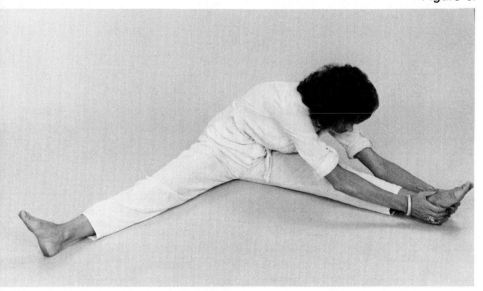

Hip Pushups

Continue with HIP PUSHUPS. Assume a prone position, toes supporting your lower body, with your hands under your face and your elbows out to the sides so that most of your weight rests on your forearms. (Figure 7.) Lift your torso and legs completely off the floor. Now, push up at the hips until you are balanced on your toes and forearms and your body forms a triangle. (Figure 8.) Hold this position for a count of three. Release so that you are lying relaxed on the floor. Rest for a count of two. Do five repetitions. This is less difficult than a conventional pushup, but it is still very effective in building strength through your neck and back and in straightening out your back.

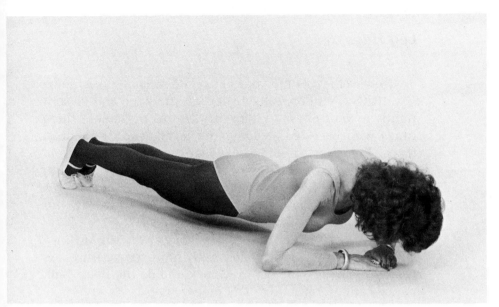

Figure 7.

Figure 8.

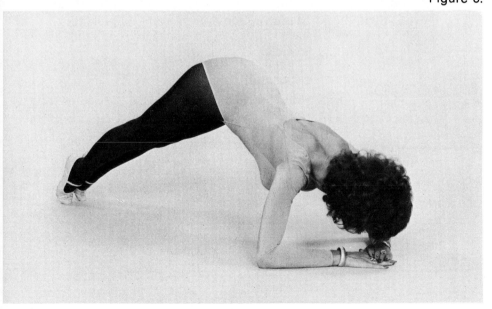

Leg Hugs

Now, roll over onto your back. You're going to do some LEG HUGS. Bend one of your legs at the knee and clasp it tightly to your chest. (Figure 9.) Do this movement three times with each leg, holding the position for a count of three. Relax for three counts, then press again. Now repeat the exercise, this time clasping both knees with both arms. (Figure 10.) Repeat for a total of four times. This not only strengthens your arm and thigh muscles, but presses down and straightens out your back.

The exercises you do for your back will pay off in a stronger, more flexible back and improved posture. As time goes by, take a Posture Check and do the Book Walk periodically to measure your improvement.

Also help your back as well as your posture by doing the Partial Pushups of Chapter 3, the Hail Hero, Cobra and Yoga Sit of Chapter 6, the Pushups of Chapter 10, and the Seated and Standing Toe Touches of Chapter 12.

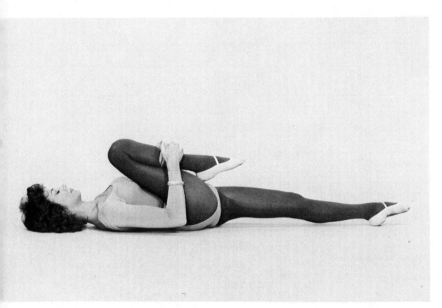

Figure 9.

Figure 10.

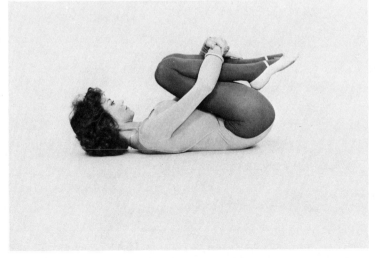

10
THE BUST

THE BUST LINE is a cause for concern for more women than is any other part of their bodies, with the possible exception of their derrières or hips. A few of the Hollywood stars still fake a bit more bust than is theirs by nature, but scanty modern dress, especially evening gowns and bikinis, leaves little to the imagination and generally requires honesty. Breast enhancement is one of the most common forms of modern cosmetic surgery. Whether you go that route is up to you. But first try natural development. Just as some women, especially in Beverly Hills, go to plastic surgeons seeking a nose like Pam Dawber's or a bust like Dolly Parton's, women came to me with the desire to enlarge their bust lines through exercise. One attractive but tiny lady all but demanded Dollylike dimensions. If she had offered me millions, I couldn't have achieved that for her. And if I could have, she'd never have been able to stand up straight! The truth is being overly endowed has its problems. Top-heavy women often suffer from unwanted male attention and find their ample proportions a physical burden as well. If you have a lot up on top, you should do those exercises that strengthen the pectoral without enlarging the bust. If you want a larger bust, you should do the exercises that firm but include also others that will tend to enlarge your breasts. No matter what size bust you have, you should develop it in proportion with the rest of you. A woman, especially a small woman, can have a fine shape even with a small bust if her breasts are firm.

Circular Arm Swings

While I do not normally advocate power exercises, for developing the bust line I find them as beneficial as stretching exercises. However, such exercises impose a lot of strain on your heart, so take it easy if you are not in top condition. Let's begin by working with weights — perhaps books or dumbbells — of no more than three to four pounds each: just enough to add stress. Try these CIRCULAR ARM SWINGS. Stand comfortably with your feet 12 to 18 inches apart. Grip a weight in each hand. Raise your arms up and out to the sides (Figure 1), then swing them down until they cross (Figure 2), and continue the swing up until you are holding your arms at about shoulder level. (Figure 3.) Bring them back down, uncrossing them, and follow through in one continuous movement until your arms are stretched out to the sides, then repeat. Do ten arm swings consecutively but slowly, stressing the stretch in the third phase (as you uncross your arms and bring them back up to the outstretched position). This exercise not only will build up, firm up, and tone up your breast muscles, but will work wonders for the flab that tends to develop under your upper arms.

Figure 1.

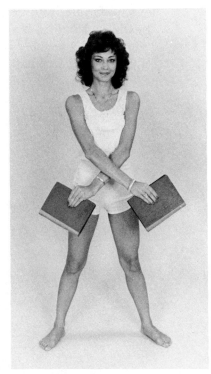

Figure 2.

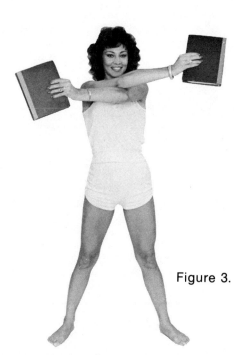

Figure 3.

PARTS OF THE BODY

Weight Pushes

Now, lie on your back, on the floor if you wish, but preferably across a bench or two stools that permit your legs to dangle from bent knees, with toes barely touching the floor. Holding a weight in each hand, drop your elbows down so that the weights are level with your chest (Figure 4), then push your arms straight overhead. (Figure 5.) Repeat this movement ten times, slowly but continuously. Inhale deeply through your nose as you push the weights up, and exhale through your mouth as you bring them down.

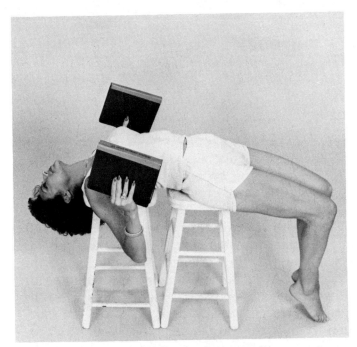

Figure 4.

Figure 5.

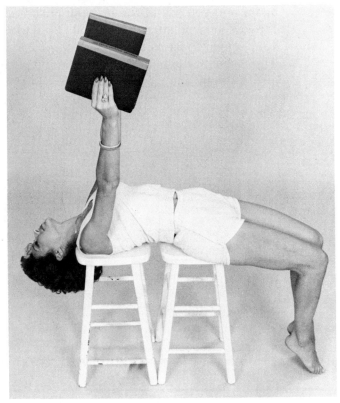

PARTS OF THE BODY

Arm Strokes

Moving on from weights, let's do ARM STROKES. This exercise is similar to the breast stroke in swimming — which, by the way, is wonderful for developing the chest, the pectoral muscles, the shoulder muscles, and the arm muscles. Stand with your feet about 12 inches apart. Bend your arms so that your elbows are out to the sides at shoulder height and the fingertips of both hands touch in front of you. (Figure 6.) Pull your hands away from each other until your fingertips point straight ahead of you and your elbows are pointing straight back. (Figure 7.) In your imagination try to make your shoulder blades touch each other. Now, bring your fingertips together until they touch again and you are in the original position. Do twenty Arm Strokes in rapid succession. You should feel tension across your upper chest as you draw your arms all the way back. This primarily benefits your chest and pectoral muscles. It also tightens the shoulder muscles.

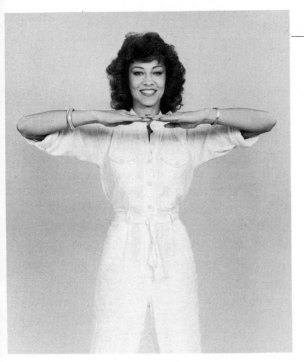

Figure 6.

Figure 7.

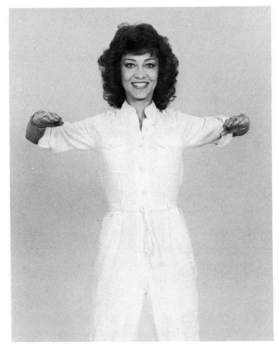

PARTS OF THE BODY

Arm Isometrics

If you want to add a few power developments, try ARM ISOMETRICS. Clasp the fingers of one hand around the wrist of the other so that your arms are locked together, then try to pull them apart. (Figure 8.) Next, place your palms together and press them hard against each other. (Figure 9.) These exercises develop many of the upper body muscles as well as helping to enlarge the bust.

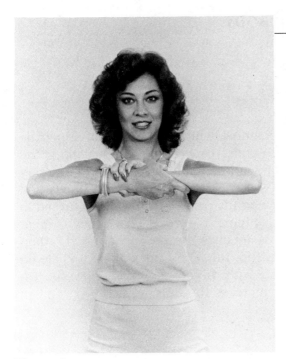

Figure 8.

Figure 9.

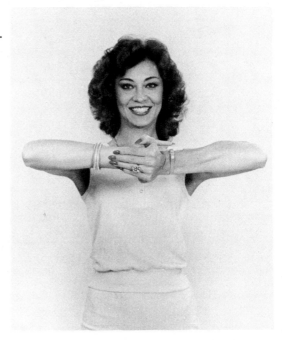

Modified Pushups

Now for some pushups, which can be demanding to do but are very worthwhile, especially for developing the bust, back, shoulders, and arms. It's only really necessary to do MODIFIED PUSHUPS. Get down on your hands and knees on the floor, with the palms of your hands turned in toward each other. (Figure 10.) Slowly lower your upper body until your nose touches the floor (Figure 11), then slowly push yourself up. Inhale on the way up, exhale on the way down. Start with three pushups in slow succession and gradually increase the number to six.

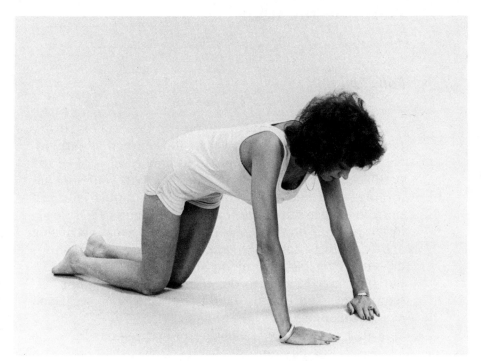

Figure 10.

Figure 11.

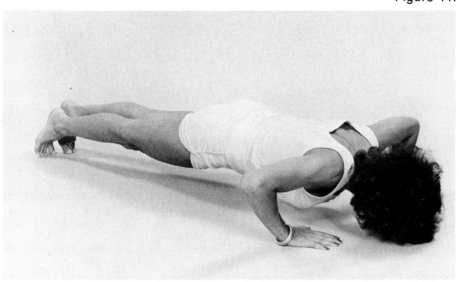

PARTS OF THE BODY

Full Pushups

If you want to go further, you can do FULL PUSHUPS. Lie flat on the floor, with your palms turned slightly inward and your elbows pointed out to the sides. (See the position of the arms in Figure 11.) Using your toes for leverage and keeping your legs straight, push yourself until your arms are fully extended. (Figure 12.) Slowly lower yourself down to the floor. Try to avoid collapsing and lying there for long periods after each one. Pushups are great exercise for building up every part of your body, but they are difficult to do. If you're feeling strong, attempt three Full Pushups and try to build up to six. Don't overdo this one.

Other exercises you can do to improve your bust line are the Partial Pushups of Chapter 3, the Hip Pushups of Chapter 9, and the Weight Swings, Towel Twists and Shoulder Shrugs of Chapter 11.

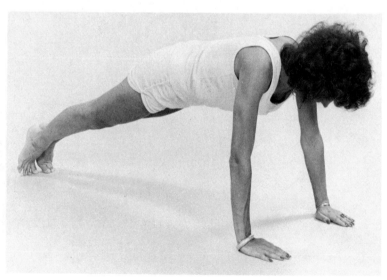

Figure 12.

11

THE SHOULDERS AND ARMS

NO ONE HAS ASKED ME yet to build up her upper body to resemble Arnold Schwarzenegger's or Martina Navratilova's. Few women want full muscular development across their shoulders and through their arms. The purpose here is to develop your muscles so that you will have good posture and a firm bust line and to tone and firm your muscles so you are strong enough to do those physical things you want to do. The trick, then, is to be very selective in choosing exercises to give you the results you want while skipping those power exercises that female body-builders use to work out.

We want curves in the right places, of course, but what we are really striving for is the long, slender look. Today, the Joan Crawford look is out. The Jayne Mansfield or Marilyn Monroe look is out. The Brooke Shields look is in, but we can't all look like teen-agers. We can only try, as the years go by, not to drift too far from our teen-age bodies. In my case, as I mentioned before, I didn't have one until ten years later.

More Weight Swings

Back to the books. Let's begin with some WEIGHT SWINGS, using books or dumbbells of three to four pounds. Grandma used the label "goose skin" for that loose skin that tends to hang down from the lower part of the upper arms. The fact is, it would have to be a fat goose, because what is hanging there is fat and soft muscle. You have to tighten and develop that muscle if you want to look good in swimsuits or short-sleeved blouses. This exercise is wonderful for those upper arms as well as for the shoulder and chest muscles. Holding a weight in each hand, bend over from the waist, keeping your back straight and flat. Your arms should be close to your sides and bent at the elbows. Now, raise the elbows, hold (Figure 1), then straighten your arms, swinging them as far up and back as you can. (Figure 2.) Hold. Then swing your arms forward and hold. (This position is not illustrated.) Drop your arms down and relax. Then repeat. Hold each position for a count of three and relax for a count of three. Start with five repetitions and build up to ten.

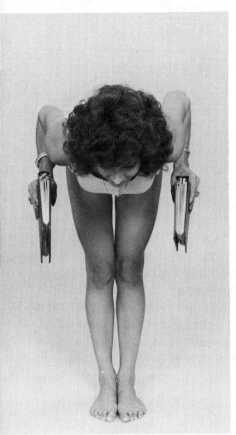

Figure 1.

Figure 2.

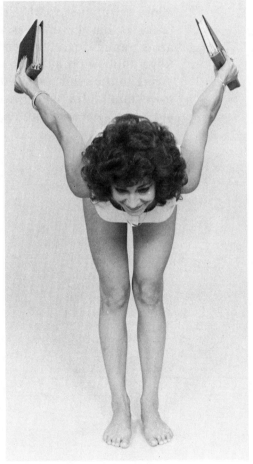

119

Towel Twists

Now, let's reach for a towel. You can use a yardstick or straight rod of any sort if you wish, but I prefer a towel. You have to pull it tightly to keep it straight, but that in itself does wonders for your arms, shoulders, and chest. Basically, TOWEL TWISTS are wonderful for the arms, shoulders, waist, and hips. Stand straight with your feet about 16 inches apart. Grip an end of the towel in each hand so that the towel is stretched tight. Now, raise your arms straight over your head (Figure 3) and, keeping the towel taut, bend at the waist to one side (Figure 4), then swing to the other side. (Figure 5.) Remember to keep the towel taut all the way. Swing easily back and forth to each side five times. Gradually increase to ten side-to-side swings.

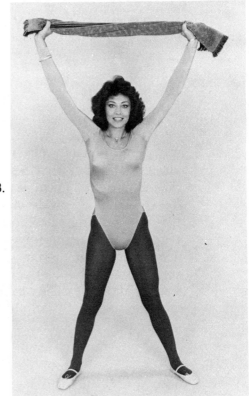

Figure 3.

Figure 4.

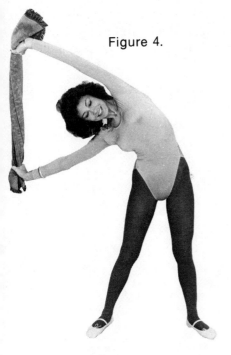

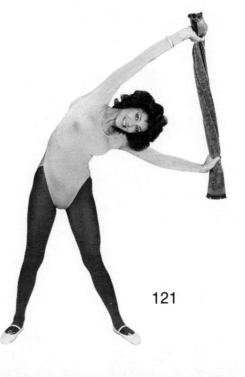

Figure 5.

PARTS OF THE BODY

Towel Swings

Next, TOWEL SWINGS. Still standing with legs well apart, pull that taut towel high to one side with one arm straight and the other bent, as if you were holding up a flag. (Figure 6.) Then swing the towel down, around, and back on the other side of your body. (Figure 7.) Repeat, this time starting with the other arm. This simple exercise tends to tighten the upper arms, the backs of the upper arms, and the forearms, and to increase the free movement of the shoulders. Both these towel exercises are wonderful for flexibility in the upper body and in the hips. They are especially helpful for those people who play golf or tennis.

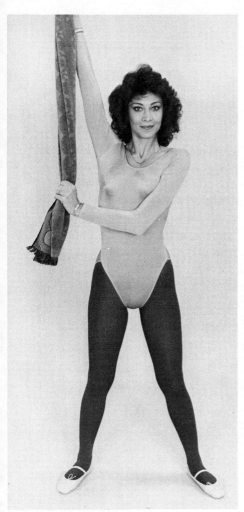

Figure 6.

Figure 7.

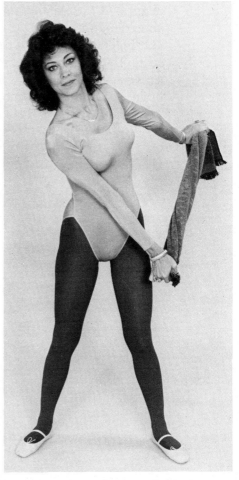

123

PARTS OF THE BODY

Shoulder Shrugs

An activity that works wonders for the shoulders and neck, SHOULDER SHRUGS do much more for you than you'd expect because they are so easy. However, you have to do them right. Stand straight with your feet slightly apart. Arms at your sides, draw your shoulders back as far as you can, and pull your stomach in as far as you can. (Figure 8.) Hold for a count of three. Then draw your shoulders and chest up, arch your head back (Figure 9), and hold for a count of three. In Figure 9, I am drawn up so tautly that you can see my ribs through my leotard. This exercise doubles as a rib cage lift. Do five at first and build up to ten at a time.

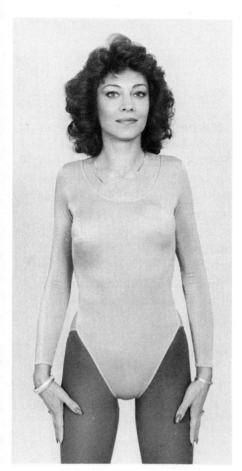

Figure 8.

Figure 9.

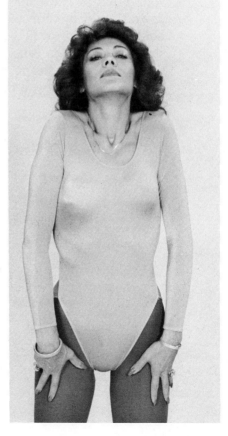

Rib Cage Raises

Now, let's do some RIB CAGE RAISES, which are super for the arms and shoulders as well as the waistline. This exercise also develops flexibility. Stand as straight as you can with legs well apart. Lace your fingers together, then raise your arms over your head so that the palms of your hands are turned up toward the ceiling. (Figure 10.) Reach as high as you can, lifting your rib cage. Hold for a count of five. Now, still keeping your rib cage up, bend your arms at the elbows and bring your clasped hands down right over your head. Press your palms together and hold for a count of five. (Figure 11.) Done with as much stretch as possible, this movement lifts the breasts, trims the waist, straightens and strengthens the back, and stretches and firms up the arm muscles. Do five complete Rib Cage Raises.

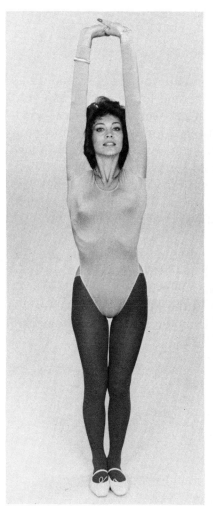

Figure 10.

Figure 11.

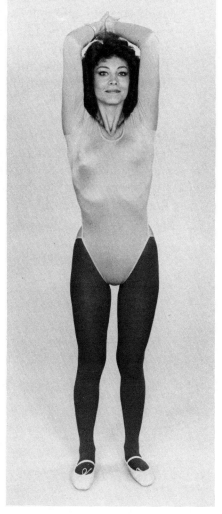

Arm Stretches

Lastly, ARM STRETCHES. With your legs spread 12 to 18 inches apart to give you a solid foundation, clasp your hands behind your back as if in a soldier's "at ease" position. Now, bend forward from your waist, keeping your back straight and flat, and swing your arms back above your head. (Figure 12.) Hold for a count of three. Then, straighten up, unclasp and drop your hands, and relax. Repeat this exercise for a total of five times. Stretch out, back, and up as much as you can. Stretch, stretch, stretch.

Also beneficial for the shoulders and arms are the Arm-Leg Hugs of Chapter 1, the Partial Pushups of Chapter 3, the Hand Reaches and Hip Pushups of Chapter 9, the Circular Arm Swings and the Pushups of Chapter 10, the Elbow Twist Situps of Chapter 12, and the Rear End Rocks of Chapter 13.

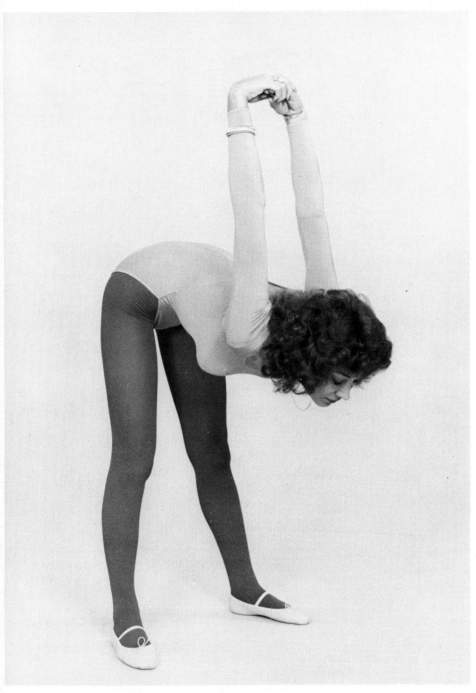

Figure 12.

12
THE WAIST AND ABDOMEN

LIKE THE LADY WHO WANTED to lose weight without giving up her beer, we all want to get something without giving up anything. We all like to eat — usually the wrong things. Many of us like to drink. I'm personally big on healthy diets, but that's another book. I have nothing against good food. Some of the finest restaurants in the world are found in Beverly Hills — Chasen's, which is President and Mrs. Reagan's favorite; The Bistro, La Scala, L'Escoffier, La Chaumiere, Chambord, Trader Vic's. With such riches the temptation to overeat all but does in many people. They take it in and ask me to take it off!

Well, most of us have a weight problem. I had mine early. I still don't feel as if I have it licked, as slender as I am now. I know that if I start overeating again and stop exercising I'll lose my shape fast. You have to work at losing weight. You have to work to keep it off. You have to cut back on the calories. And you have to exercise. If you all but stopped eating, you would become slender, of course. But if your muscles were not toned up, long and firm, stretched and flexible, you still would not have the attractive figure you want.

The waist and abdomen are the areas that trouble most women the most. So, let's get to work!

Standing Toe Touches

Let's begin with some STANDING TOE TOUCHES. Stand erect with your feet 12 to 18 inches apart. Raise your arms and spread them wide. (Figure 1.) Then, keeping your legs straight and pivoting from the hips, bend over and swing your right arm over and down to your left foot. (Figure 2.) Stand up again with your arms outstretched, then bend and reach your left arm to touch your right foot, trying to touch your fingertips to your toes in each case. Move continuously, alternating your arms, touching each foot five times. This action slims your waistline and tightens and trims your abdomen. It also is beneficial for the buttocks, back, shoulders, and thighs. You will receive the same benefits from the following exercise.

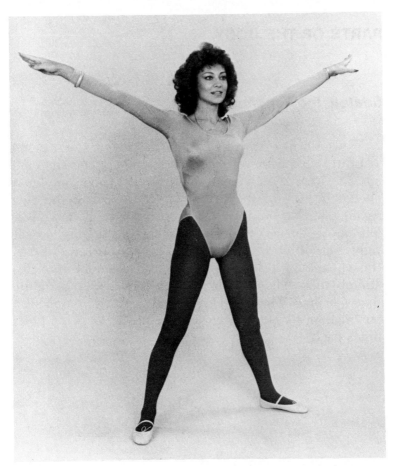

Figure 1.

Figure 2.

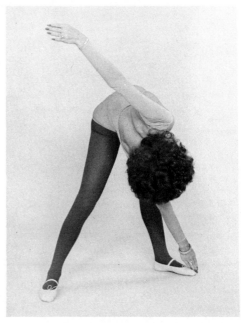

Seated Toe Touches

Now, drop into a seated position for SEATED TOE TOUCHES. Sit with your legs as straight as possible and spread as far to each side as you can get them; the knees should be toward the ceiling, not out toward the side. Again, alternate, your right fingers reaching to touch your left toes (Figure 3), and your left fingers reaching for your right toes. (Figure 4.) Stretch as far as you can to loosen those back muscles, stretch those shoulder muscles, stretch those abdomen and thigh muscles, and tighten that waistline. This exercise should be done in a continuous motion, touching each toe five times. Work up to ten times each.

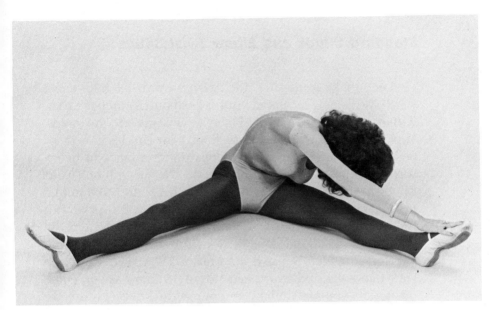

Figure 3.

Figure 4.

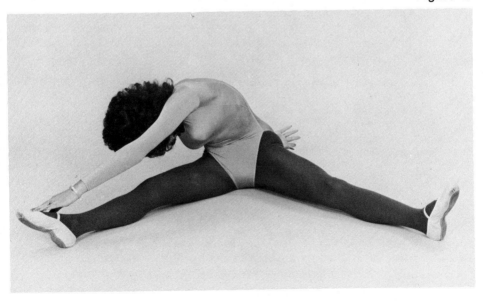

Standard Situps and Elbow Twist Situps

Let's make it tougher. Lie down on your back for some STANDARD SITUPS. Spread your legs about 18 inches apart, with your knees straight. Place your arms at your sides. You might want someone to hold your ankles down, or possibly you can hook your ankles under a piece of heavy furniture to hold them down. Now, rise up to touch your fingertips to your toes, using your back and abdominal muscles to bring you up. This is tough, of course, but there is nothing more beneficial for your abdomen. To make it easier, bend your knees. To make it tougher still, and for an added flourish, do ELBOW TWIST SITUPS. Clasp your hands behind your head (Figure 5), and as you come up, touch your left elbow to your right knee (Figure 6), and then your right elbow to your left knee. (Figure 7.) These Elbow Twist Situps are hard to do, but they do a lot for you. Do five in each position, moving continuously.

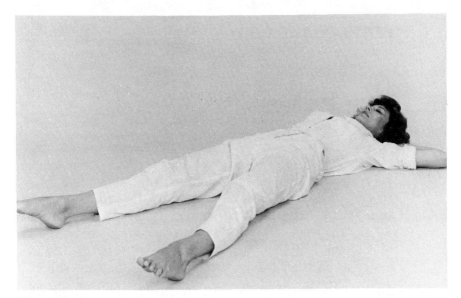

Figure 5.

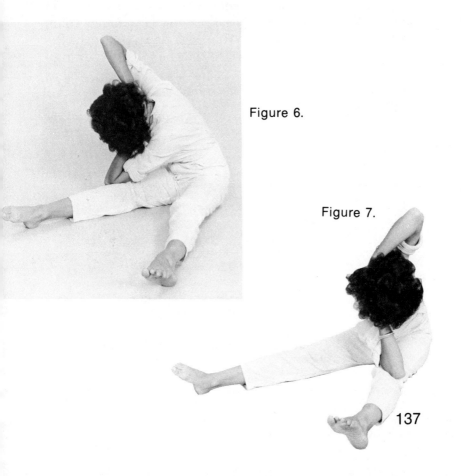

Figure 6.

Figure 7.

137

Seated Leg Raises

Now, let's do some Leg Raises. There are several ways to do these. In one version you can lie flat on your back, keeping your legs straight, and use your abdominal muscles to raise your legs 12 inches off the ground. Lower your legs slowly, then raise them again. Do five raises. Again, it is easier if your hands are at your sides, harder if they are clasped behind your head. SEATED LEG RAISES are easier to do than the lying-down version but are still effective. Sit on the floor or on a bed, a chair, or a stool. First, raise your knees, with toes pointed, and hold for a count of three. (Figure 8.) Then, extend your legs straight and lift them about 12 inches, holding for another count of three. (Figure 9.) Bring your legs down and rest. Repeat the Seated Leg Raises five times, increasing eventually to ten. These will do a lot for your thighs as well as your waist and abdomen.

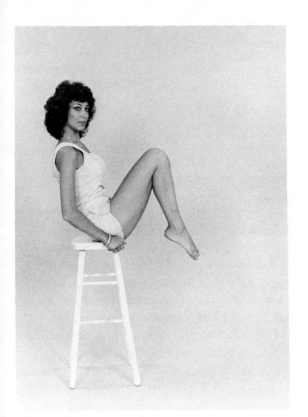

Figure 8.

Figure 9.

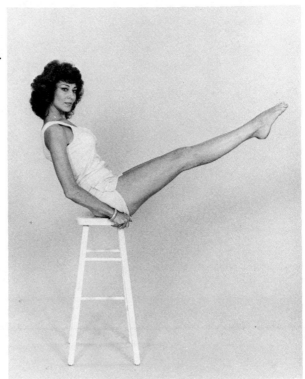

Yoga Leg Raises

On to a YOGA LEG RAISE. Lie flat on your back, hands by your sides; then, keeping your legs straight, slowly lift them up (Figure 10) and back over your head, raising your hips as you go until you are lying on your upper back and shoulders and looking up at your knees. (Figure 11.) Some of you will not be able to go all the way over, at least for a while, but go as far as you can. Do this exercise in one slow, flowing motion, and hold at the extreme position for a count of five. Then slowly lower your legs to the floor, trying to feel one vertebra at a time coming in contact with the floor. Inhale on the way up, exhale on the way down. Start with five repetitions, building to ten.

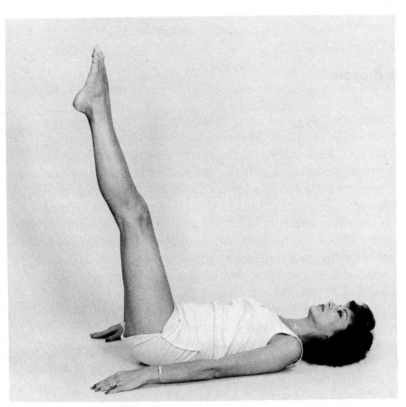

Figure 10.

Figure 11.

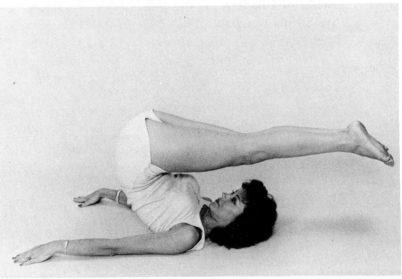

The Bicycle

From the previous exercise, you can flow smoothly into the BICYCLE. Raise and hold your derrière at the hips. Extend your legs and move them up, around, and down as if you were pedaling a bicycle. (Figures 12 and 13.) Keep your legs moving briskly for a count of twenty; rest, and repeat twice. It is important to get a full extension of your leg in the up position, a full bend at the knee in the down position. This exercise will trim down your waistline and abdomen, firm your buttocks, and do a lot for your legs. You soon will be on your way to a flatter stomach and a smaller waist.

Also good for the stomach and waist are the Sit-Reaches of Chapter 1, the Rotations and Arm Scissors of Chapter 2, the Side and Back Leg Extensions of Chapter 3, the Seated Horizontal Scissors Kick and Seated Leg Extensions of Chapter 5, the Rotation Stretches of Chapter 7, the Leg Hugs of Chapter 9, the Weight Swings and Towel Twists of Chapter 11, the Side Bends of Chapter 16, and the Situps of Chapter 17.

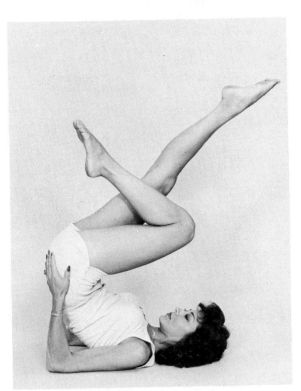

Figure 12.

Figure 13.

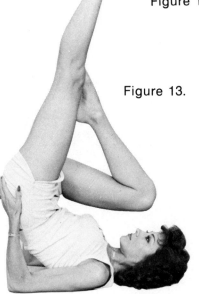

13

THE HIPS AND BUTTOCKS

NOTHING IS MORE unflattering than a large derrière. When I gain weight, it shows up behind me first. I don't have to look at it, but others do. Lots of you who think you look pretty good in slacks or jeans should see yourselves as others see you.

You're not alone, you know. A lot of curvy screen stars, some of whom were my clients, find their figures betraying them from behind and have to work hard to keep their curves in proportion. A firm fanny is greatly to be desired. But not easily attained. Normally we neglect these muscles. If we sit a lot, perhaps at a desk at work, we develop that miserable malady known as "secretary's spread." In our everyday activities we do not tighten and trim the derrière, so let's go at it now.

The Tush Press

Start by simply pressing in firmly with a hand on each side of your buttocks (Figure 1), tensing the muscles in your buttocks. Hold for a count of five. Relax and grab again, perhaps in a slightly different position. I call this the TUSH PRESS. It is also helpful to simply tighten up your buttocks and hold for a count of five. An offbeat but highly effective exercise was suggested by the people at The Fashion Academy in Costa Mesa. Place a quarter between your cheeks, not too far in, and walk around awhile. You will have to maintain tension in your buttocks to keep the quarter in place.

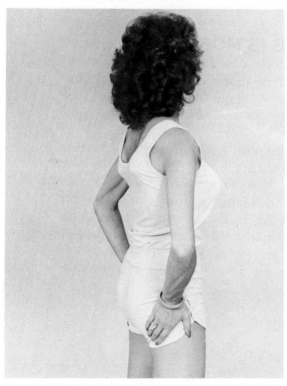

Figure 1.

Rear Leg Raises

REAR LEG RAISES are really effective in trimming the tush, provided you push each leg to its full extension and raise it high behind you. Stand where you can hold onto something for balance and push your leg back and up behind you. (Figure 2.) Alternate legs ten times each and hold each leg up for a count of ten. Again, this simple exercise can be done not only while working out, but also at the filing cabinet or at the sink. This is good for the entire leg, too.

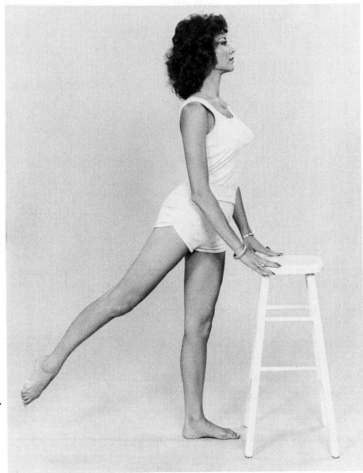

Figure 2.

Crossover Side Kicks

CROSSOVER SIDE KICKS provide a strong pull on the posterior, firm the thighs, and develop flexibility in the hips. With one hand balanced on a chair, desk, dresser, sink, or whatever, and the other hand on your hip, hold your outside leg off the ground and out to the side. (Figure 3.) Cross your outside leg over your inside leg, swinging it to full extension, and hold for a count of five. (Figure 4.) Repeat this movement ten times, swinging continuously. Concentrate on getting full extension with your leg. Then, turn to face the other direction and repeat with the other leg.

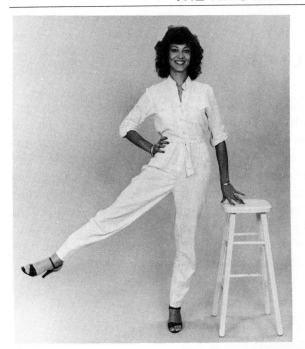

Figure 3.

Figure 4.

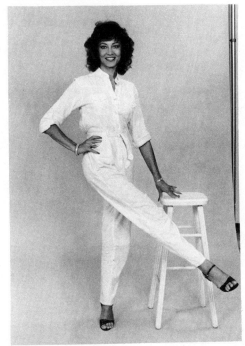

Rear End Rock

Drop down to a seated position for a little REAR END ROCK. Sit with your knees out to the side and the soles of your feet pressed together, your hands clasping your ankles. (Figure 5.) Now, simply rock from side to side (Figure 6) continuously and hard, trying to press your knees toward the floor while lifting from side to side with your thighs, hips, and buttocks. You should feel a strong pull in your buttocks and thighs, even in your shoulders and arms. This will take weight off your derrière and hips while stretching and toning the muscles there.

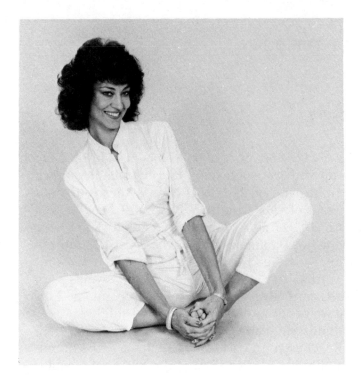

Figure 5.

Figure 6.

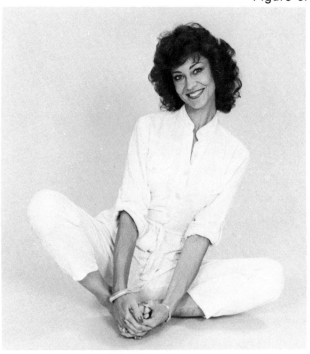

Side Scissors

Time to relax. Sort of. Lie on your left side, holding your head up with your left hand and balancing yourself with your right hand on the floor. Now, swing your right leg out in front of you. (Figure 7.) Swing it back behind you. (Figure 8.) Do in a continuous motion. Keep your knee straight, toes pointed, and work at getting full extension with your leg. Do ten SIDE SCISSORS with your right leg. Turn to the other side and do ten swings with the left leg. Eventually work up to twenty repetitions. This works very well for the derrière, hips, and thighs.

Other things you can do for the hips and derrière are the Hand Reaches and Leg Hugs of Chapter 9, the Standing Toe Touches of Chapter 12, and the Situps of Chapter 17.

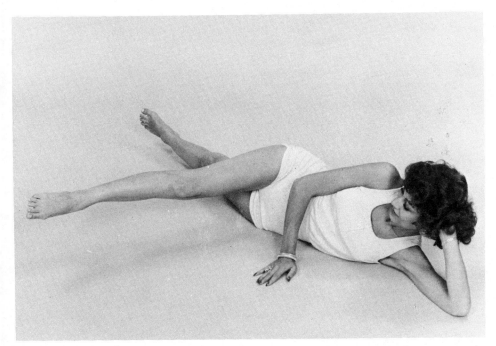

Figure 7.

Figure 8.

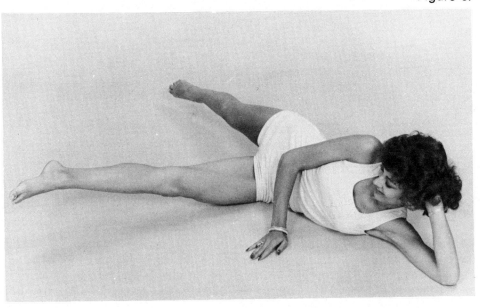

14
THE THIGHS

WE ARE self-conscious about our thighs in sunny Southern California, where we wear shorts and swimsuits so much of the time. Many women who look trim on top look terrible from the waist down, and when they bare their thighs, they betray their worst-kept secret.

Thighs ranked with the bust and derrière as priority items among many of my clients, especially the older women who were remaining in show business. Dancers build big, muscular thighs. They can't help that, but they also stretch their thigh muscles to lengthen them. They have to work to keep them in shape. Even if you've danced your last dance, you will want to work to tighten and lengthen those thighs.

PARTS OF THE BODY

Side Leg Extensions

Start with some SIDE LEG EXTENSIONS. Stand with your palm flat on some surface for balance. Swing your outer leg out to the side as far as possible, keeping your leg as straight as possible and flexing your foot at the ankle so that the sole of your foot is parallel to the floor. (Figure 1.) Feel the pull through your thighs. Bring your leg back, but do not touch the floor. (Figure 2.) Do ten Side Leg Extensions. Then face in the other direction and repeat with the other leg.

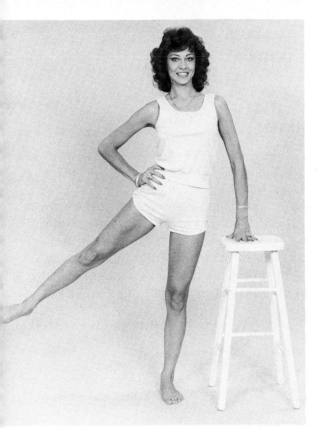

Figure 2.

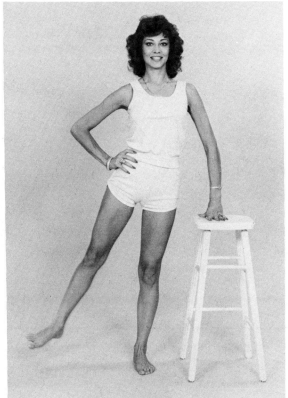

PARTS OF THE BODY

Front Leg Extensions

Now, let's do FRONT LEG EXTENSIONS. This is the same exercise except that the action is in front of you. Stand with one hand resting on a convenient surface for balance. (Figure 3.) Concentrate on getting full extension of your leg and foot as you raise your leg directly in front of you until you can feel the tension in the thigh muscle. (Figure 4.) Keep the knees of both legs straight. Hold each raise for a count of five. Do ten Front Leg Extensions with each leg.

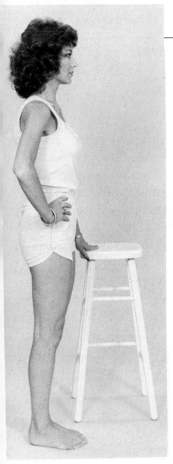

Figure 3.

Figure 4.

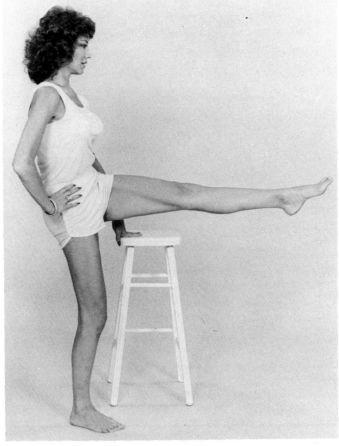

Leg Lunges

Move on to LEG LUNGES. These are more advanced than they may seem, so start slowly. Standing up straight, hands on your lower hips, lunge to one side, bending your knee, while extending the other leg straight. (Figure 5.) Return to the standing position, pushing yourself upright with your knee. Then, lunge to the other side. (Figure 6.) Move continuously but slowly, pushing from one side to the other ten times — five times to each side. If you feel tension in both thighs, you are doing the exercise properly. This is also good for the calves, ankles, and feet.

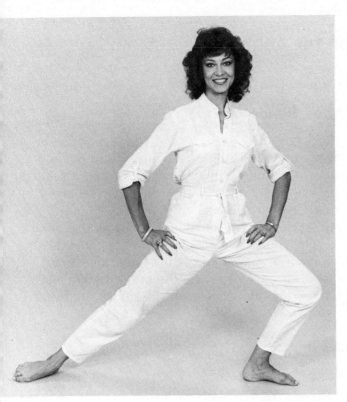

Figure 5.

Figure 6.

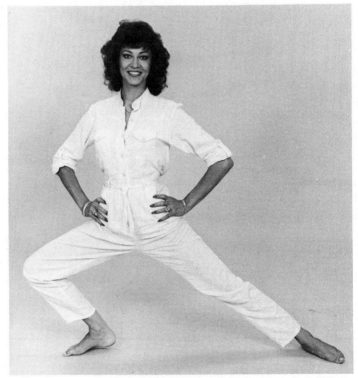

Halfway Knee Bends

I do not recommend full knee bends; they put too much stress on the knee. But HALFWAY KNEE BENDS do the job of stressing the thighs. Stand with your feet about 18 inches apart, with your hands on your hips. (Figure 7.) Keeping your back straight and buttocks tucked under, press down with your knees pointing out to the sides. (Figure 8.) Come up, then down again — ten times in all. Press down just far enough to feel the pull through your thighs each time. This also is good for the ankles and feet.

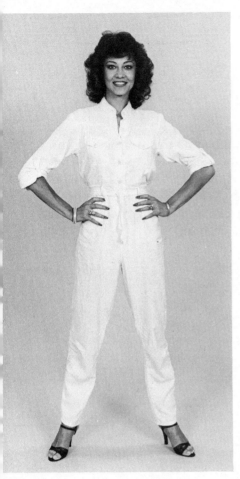

Figure 7.

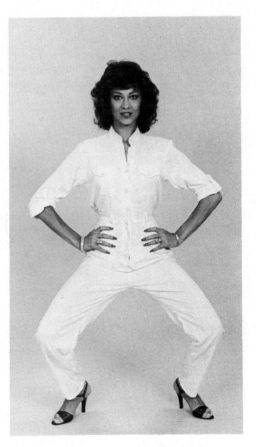

Figure 8.

Back Stretches

Kneel down now, with your arms outstretched (Figure 9) for some BACK STRETCHES. Lean back as though pulling on a rope (Figure 10), but not so far that you force your knees into a total bend. Keep your back straight and lean back until you feel a strong pull through your thighs. Slowly return to an upright position.

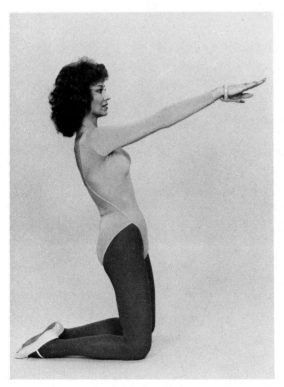

Figure 9.

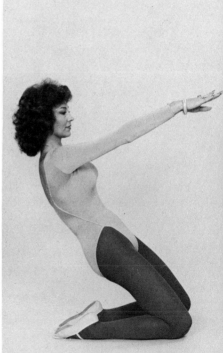

Figure 10.

164

The Bicycle

Back to the BICYCLE. I don't want to repeat too many exercises, but this one is super for the thighs as well as the waist. Lie on your back and raise up your legs and hips. Support your hips with your hands and move your legs up, around, and down in a bicycling motion. (Figure 11.) Remember to fully extend your legs and fully bend your knees as you circle. Real bicycling itself is good for the thighs. Don't be afraid to mix some athletic activity — tennis, golf, running, swimming, especially swimming — into your weekly routine. But if you want to benefit specific parts of your body, you will have to do specific exercises.

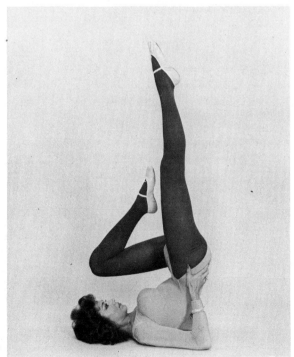

Figure 11.

Other thigh tighteners include the Alternate Leg Raises, Alternate Leg Curls, and Sit-Reaches of Chapter 1; the Reclining Leg Scissors of Chapter 2; the Side and Back Leg Extensions of Chapter 3; the Seated Leg Swings and Horizontal Scissors Kicks and Seated Leg Extensions of Chapter 5; the Hail Hero of Chapter 6; the Back Leg Extensions and Leg Hugs of Chapter 9; the Bicycle, Yoga Leg Raises, and Seated Toe Touches of Chapter 12; the Rear Leg Raises, Crossover Side Kicks, Rear End Rocks and Side Scissors of Chapter 13; and the Situps and Leg Spreads of Chapter 17.

15
THE CALVES, ANKLES, AND FEET

WHEN WE WALK BRISKLY, jog, or run, we put many pounds of pressure on our feet. Many of us are on our feet all day long. And we often put them into fancy high-heeled shoes that force our feet and arches, ankles and lower legs into extremely unnatural positions. We really do wrong by our feet. It's time we did right for them. They are badly neglected in most exercise books.

Foot Lifts

A lot of ladies, including teen-age girls, are pestered by what are called "piano legs" — thick calves and ankles that look sturdy enough to support a baby grand. FOOT LIFTS are the best thing you can do for your calves, ankles, and feet. They can be done not only during an exercise period, but while standing in line, while washing dishes at the sink, and in other standing-still situations. Simply stand up straight and rise up as high as you can on the balls and toes of your feet (Figure 1), hold for a count of five, return your heels to the floor (Figure 2), and relax. Then, repeat. This exercise can be particularly effective when done while balancing on the edge of a thick book, such as a big-city telephone book, with your weight on the balls of your feet. This way, you can not only raise yourself up, but lower yourself down, without touching your heels to the floor, an important stretching motion for your arches.

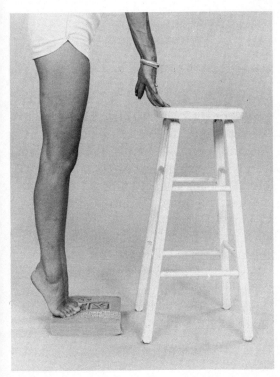

Figure 1.

Figure 2.

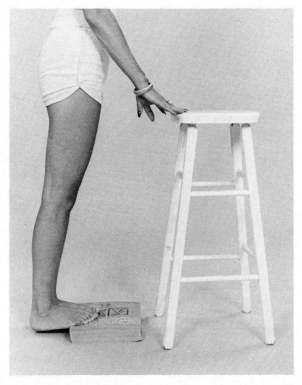

PARTS OF THE BODY

Ankle Turns

ANKLE TURNS are easy, but they are effective not only for the ankle, but also the calf and the foot. Sit down and lean back, supporting yourself with your hands. Raise and extend one leg and foot fully, stressing your thigh and calf muscles, as you pull your foot back taut (Figure 3), turning it first to one side, then to the other. (Figure 4.) Make circles in a continuous motion. Repeat for a few minutes, then switch to the other leg and foot. These Ankle Turns can be done while sitting down and talking on the phone or watching television. If you will concentrate on full extensions and do them slowly but continuously for a few minutes, they can be very effective in bringing you the beautiful legs you so much want.

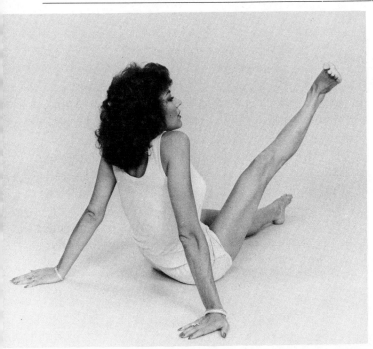

Figure 3.

Figure 4.

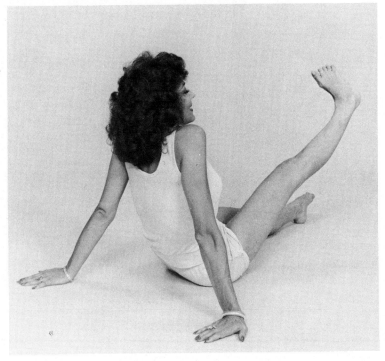

PARTS OF THE BODY

The Pencil Walk

The PENCIL WALK is an effective antidote for falling arches and really flexes the calves, ankles, and arches. Place a pencil on the floor. Now, pick it up with your toes. (Figure 5.) If your toe muscles are not strong enough to pick it up, put the pencil where your toes can grip it until they are strong enough to pick it up themselves. Walk on your heels without dropping the pencil. Now, switch the pencil to the other foot and walk again. You will not be able to walk far, but taking a few steps this way and that will work wonders for your lower legs and feet.

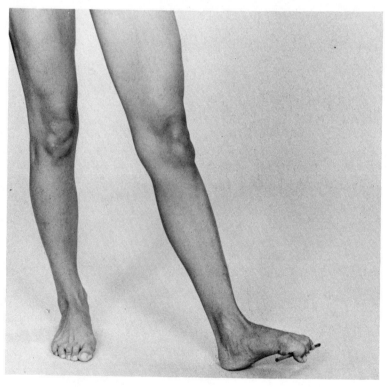

Figure 5.

THE CALVES, ANKLES, AND FEET

Walking itself is a wonderful exercise for the feet, ankles, calves, and thighs. If you walk far enough, briskly enough to get good circulation going throughout your body, you will benefit enormously. I am not a great advocate of jogging or running. It is fine for those conditioned to it, but it stresses and strains the joints too much. Personally, I believe you would be better off with a combination of the specialized calisthenic exercises in this book, brisk walking, and perhaps some sporting activity.

Additional activities for your calves, ankles, and feet would be the Alternate Leg Raises and Alternate Leg Curls of Chapter 1, the Seated Leg Extensions and Foot Lifts of Chapter 5, the Back Leg Extensions of Chapter 9, the Bicycle of Chapter 12, the Rear Leg Raises of Chapter 13, and the Leg Lunges and Halfway Knee Bends of Chapter 14.

PART THREE

SOME-THING SPECIAL

16
DAYS OFF

ONE OF THE BEAUTIFUL things about life in Southern California is that we can live outdoors a lot the year around. It is not only the Beautiful People of Beverly Hills who have backyard swimming pools or live in round-the-pool apartment houses. We are on the ocean, near the desert, and surrounded by mountains. We can swim in summerlike heat in the morning and ski in winterlike cold in the afternoon.

If you can afford it, you might want to vacation in Beverly Hills, perhaps staying long enough to see how the Beautiful People live, to visit the fashionable shops, and to dine at the sumptuous restaurants. You might check in at the Beverly Hills Hotel, where many people meet to make deals over lunch or drinks in the Polo Lounge, and where the early-morning mist hanging over the outdoor pool by the bungalows in back will remind you of many a movie scene. There also are other places to stay if you want to bring a little glamour and elegance into your life: the Beverly Wilshire or the Beverly Hilton, or even one of the several small but swank hostelries such as Max Bariel's.

But life can be beautiful anywhere you live. And you can be beautiful. We all have time off and lovely places to visit. While having fun in the sun, do not neglect your body. Warm up properly before any athletic activity to avoid strain and pain. Stretch and loosen those muscles and joints. Take advantage of the opportunity to get in a little exercise.

Wings

Let's begin with WINGS. Standing erect, feet comfortably apart, bring your arms to chest level, fingertips touching (Figure 1), then draw them apart, spreading your arms wide like wings. (Figure 2.) Move your arms back and forth briskly between the two positions in a continuous motion for a few minutes. This action will loosen up your arm and shoulder muscles.

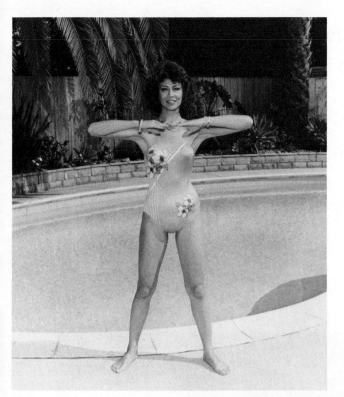

Figure 1.

Figure 2.

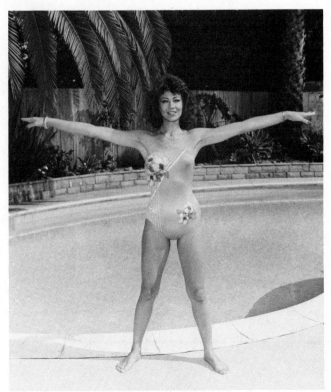

Rotations

Place your hands on your hips for some ROTATIONS. Standing with your feet well apart, bend from the waist to one side (Figure 3), then circle in a continuous motion forward (Figure 4), around to the other side, and to the back. (Figure 5.) When you have made a full circle, straighten up, then do another round. Do ten rounds in all. Concentrate on achieving full extension in every position. This exercise will loosen up your hips and back, while tightening your waist.

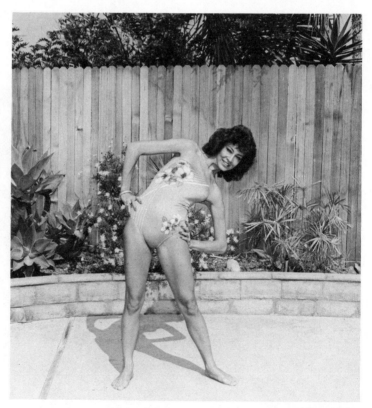

Figure 3.

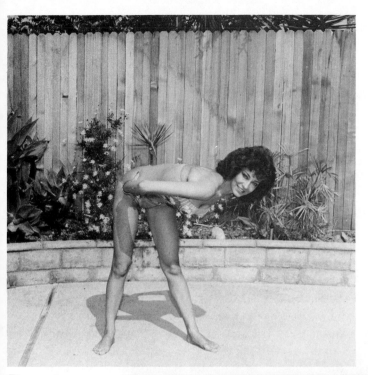

Figure 4.

Figure 5.

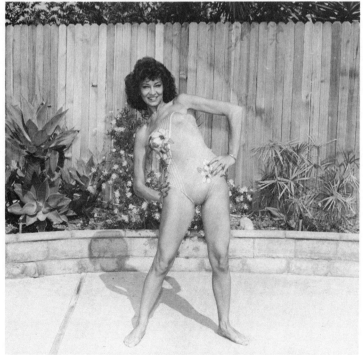

SOMETHING SPECIAL

Side Bends

Now, standing with your legs spread wide and with one arm curved over your head, bend to one side, running the hand of your other arm as far down your leg as you can reach. (Figure 6.) Bend directly to the side; don't allow your torso to lean forward. Now, bend to the other side, reaching as far down the leg on that side as possible. (Figure 7.) Stretch as fully as you can to each side as you do these SIDE BENDS to get the most from them. You should feel stress in your sides, thighs, and calves. You are stretching and toning these muscles, reducing your waistline, and warming up properly for physical activity.

Other exercises to try on your days off are the Alternate Leg Raises of Chapter 1, the Leg Extensions of Chapter 3, the Yoga Sit of Chapter 6, and the Back Leg Extensions of Chapter 9.

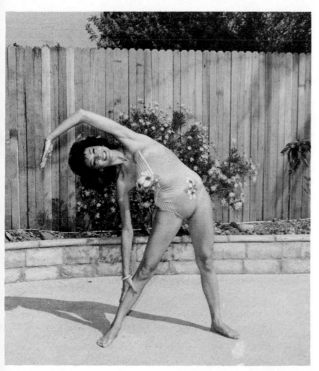

Figure 6.

Figure 7.

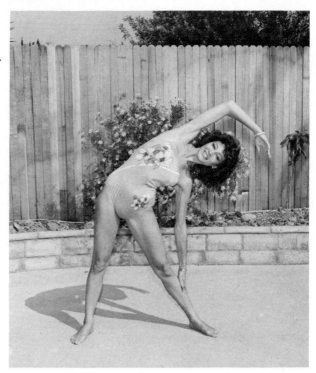

17

CHILDBIRTH

EVEN THE BEAUTIFUL People of
Beverly Hills have children. Beautiful children, of course. Childbirth doesn't have to
ruin your figure forever. I've had three children and it hasn't ruined mine. There are
exercises you can do before childbirth to prepare your
body properly and exercises you can do afterwards to restore your body to its former form — which, if you were
using this book, was pretty good. You will do some of the
same exercises both before and after, of course, because
pregnancy and childbirth make demands on a lot of the
same muscles, especially in the stomach, abdomen, and
pelvic regions.

I said in the beginning of the book that if you have any
physical problems or are not confident that you do not
have, you should check with your doctor before beginning
an exercise program. Now I want to stress that in the case
of pregnancy, you should check with your doctor about
how long before childbirth you can exercise safely, how
strenuously you can exercise, and how soon after child-

birth you can start to exercise and how strenuously. In most cases, doctors recommend exercise before and after childbirth to build up your body for the easiest possible delivery and to rebuild it for the happiest possible motherhood. With the approval of your obstetrician, let's go.

Situps

Start with SITUPS. Good old Situps. Lie flat, arms stretched to your sides, legs straight, heels tight to the floor with toes pointed. Bring your arms straight back over your head (Figure 1) and then come up and try to touch your fingertips to your toes. (Figure 2.) Keep your legs slightly bent to make it easier. If you do this before pregnancy, your abdominal muscles will be much stronger and make possible an easier delivery. Inhale on the way up, exhale on the way down. Rest in the down position for a count of three. Here, do only as many Situps as you can do comfortably. Do no more than five and fewer as you move closer toward delivery.

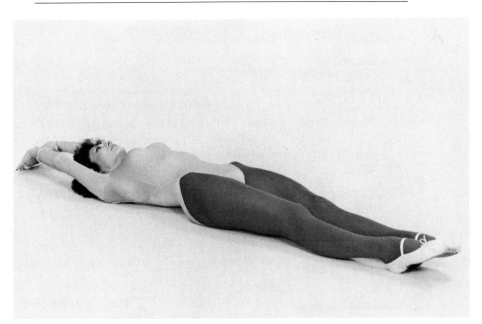

Figure 1.

Figure 2.

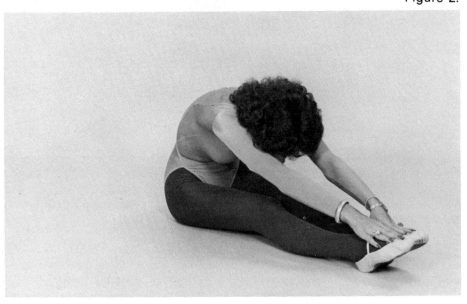

Leg Spreads

LEG SPREADS will lengthen and loosen the muscles along your inner thighs and abdomen before delivery. Begin by sitting erect and spreading your legs as far apart as you can. Bend forward and reach with your hands to hold your legs apart. (Figure 3.) But in this case do not overstretch. Come forward in a gentle rocking motion. Hold for a bit, then sit up straight again. Repeat the exercise four times, but cut back as your delivery date nears.

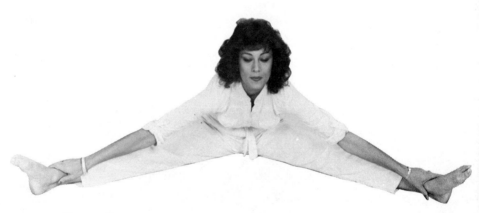

Figure 3.

188

Alternate Leg Raises

ALTERNATE LEG RAISES are excellent both before and after childbirth. You can do them briskly well before childbirth, stretching and loosening each leg. Lie on your back with your hands at your waist, then raise one leg straight overhead (Figure 4) and hold it there briefly. Lower the leg and raise your other leg. Keep a slow pace as you raise one leg and then the other. As the date draws near, do the Leg Raises more slowly. After delivery, ease back into doing this exercise. It will be beneficial in restoring tone to your stomach, abdomen, and legs.

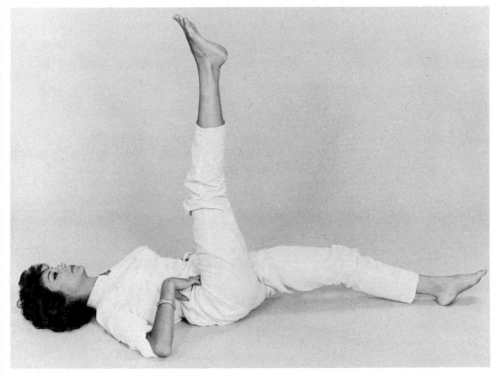

Figure 4.

Toe Pulls

The first exercise you should do after delivery is the simplest and easiest, TOE PULLS. Lie on your back, arms at your sides. Now, flex your feet toward you, keeping your heels flat to the bed or floor. Raise your head slightly to study those lovely feet (Figure 5), which soon will be moving here and there for midnight feedings and diaperings. I did this exercise in my hospital bed the day after delivery.

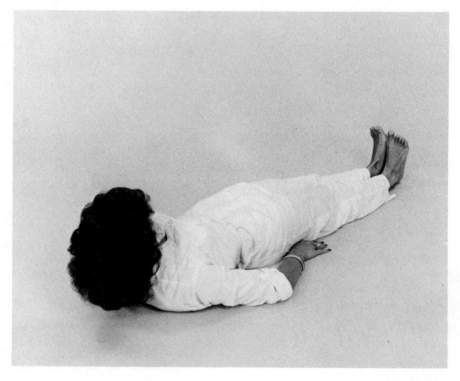

Figure 5.

Yoga Sit

After you are back home, relax with some YOGA SITS. Sit with your back straight and your knees pointing out to the sides. Press the soles of your feet together and lean forward slightly to clasp your hands comfortably in front of your feet. Gently "bounce" your knees by pushing against them with your elbows. (Figure 6.) This exercise is equally effective before and after delivery. It stretches and strengthens the principal muscles involved in childbirth and develops flexibility in your pelvic area.

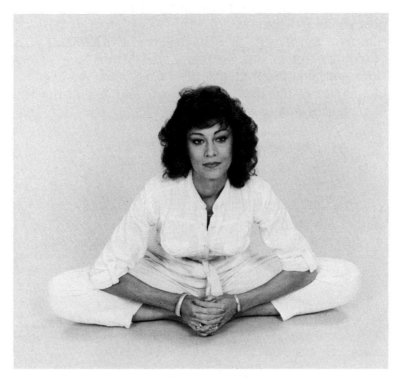

Figure 6.

Hail Hero

The good old HAIL HERO is wonderful for keeping or restoring the uterus to its proper place. Begin on your hands and knees, then reach forward and place your forearms on the floor, with elbows out to the sides and hands overlapping each other. Rest your chin on your hands. (Figure 7.) Then stretch your arms out in front of you and rock back a bit until your forehead touches the floor. Do not lower yourself onto your heels, though. (Figure 8.) The knee-to-chest position is very beneficial. It also is very restful. And after childbirth we need rest.

Other effective exercises for the pre-childbirth and post-childbirth periods are the Alternate Leg Raises, Alternate Leg Curls, and Sit-Reaches of Chapter 1, the Standing Stretches in Chapter 2, the Seated Leg Extensions and Side Leg Extensions in Chapter 3, the Yoga Sit in Chapter 6, the Cat in Chapters 7 and 9, and the Rib Cage Raises in Chapter 11.

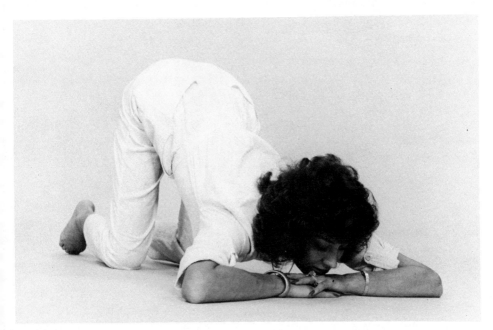

Figure 7.

Figure 8.

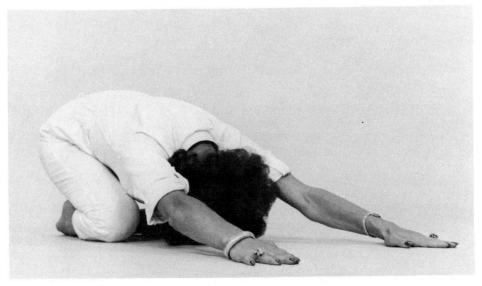

18
SHARING

MOST PEOPLE LIKE to share. With someone who cares. This is as true in Beverly Hills as it is in Boise. It is even true of exercise. Especially exercise. Done alone, as it often must be, it can be monotonous. One of the points of this book is that, taken in small doses and spread through the various activities of the day, exercise isn't too bad. But it's even better when it can be shared. With a friend. A husband. Kids. If you have any of these hanging around, enlist them in the Beverly Hills Brigade for Physical Conditioning. If you're going to be one of the Beautiful People, you want the people around you to be beautiful too. I have a husband, John. I don't have any trouble getting him to exercise; he has always been interested in physical fitness. The girls are something else, but whatever Mommy and Daddy do interests Laura, nine; Heather, six; and Christy, four. It's important to get your youngsters into the habit of exercise and physical fitness. So if you work with them, you'll be doing them a great favor. You're never too young to start. Or too old.

Togetherness Rock

John and I often join forces for a little TOGETHERNESS ROCK. Sit facing your partner, legs spread, the soles of your feet against his. Clasp hands. Now, rock back and forth. (Figure 1.) You pull him; he pulls you. (Figure 2.) John pulls me better than I pull him. But if you pull hard and resist to the point of tension, this is a terrific exercise for slimming and toning the upper torso. It stretches the shoulders, arms, back, derrière, and legs, and develops flexibility in the hips, back, and shoulders. Do at least ten pulls for each person, but don't overdo it.

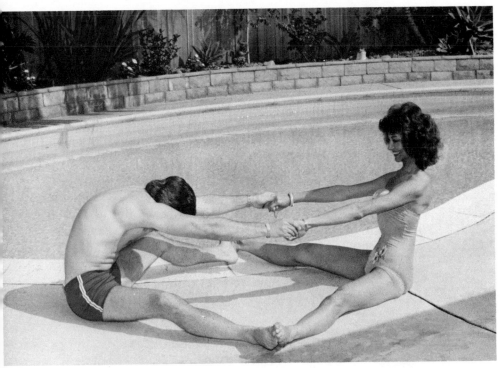

Figure 1.

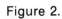
Figure 2.

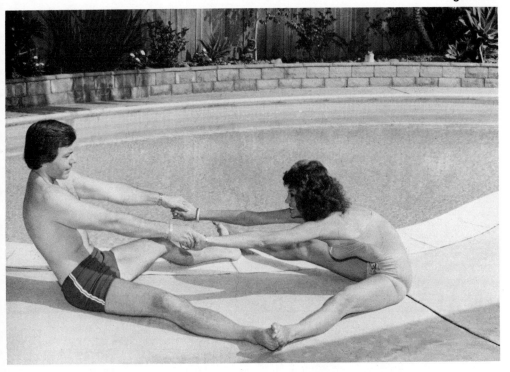

SOMETHING SPECIAL

Togetherness Twist

Now lie down on your backs, with your heads at opposite ends and your legs inside his legs so that your knees are near each other's — isn't this fun? (Figure 3.) Clasp your hands behind your heads, and do situps, turning at the waist to touch one elbow to its opposite knee, then the other elbow to its opposite knee. (Figure 4.) Return to the lying-down position and rest. Then up and at 'em again. Do five situps with fully extended twists to each side each time and build up to ten eventually. This TOGETHERNESS TWIST will trim and tone your derrière, hips, and abdomen, strengthen your legs, and make your body more flexible.

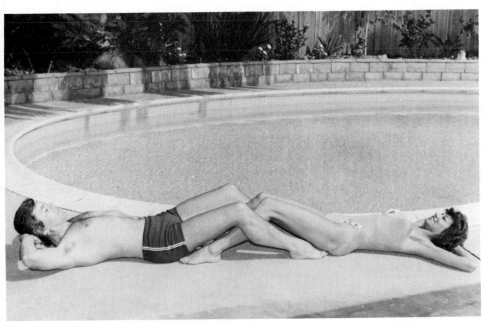

Figure 3.

Figure 4.

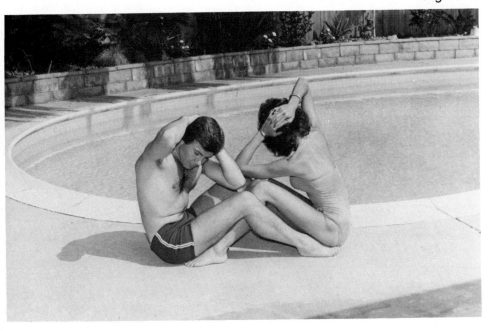

Togetherness Pushups

Finally, if the man is strong enough, he can support you in some TOGETHERNESS PUSHUPS. With your feet locked between his, lean over him and balance on his hands. (Figure 5.) Let him push you up and down. (Figure 6.) Let him do most of the work on this one. He won't mind, especially if you slip and fall. Either way, you'll benefit, too.

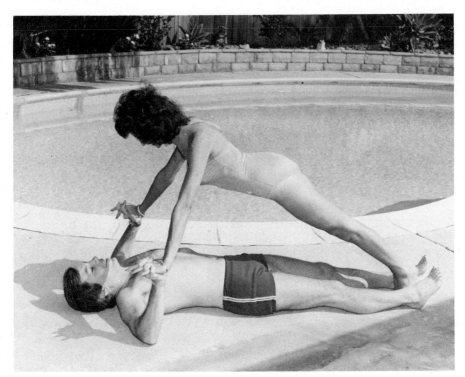

Figure 5.

Figure 6.

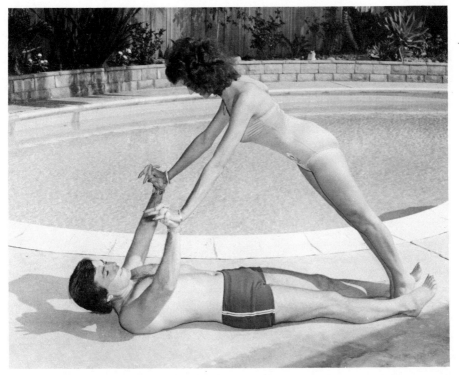

More Togetherness Twists

Now for the children. Mom and Dad can do many exercises with them, the same ones you do with your partner, or any of the other exercises. Use your imagination. Here I do more TOGETHERNESS TWISTS with one of my girls, Laura. Facing each other, legs spread, feet sole to sole — sole-mates? — arms outstretched and hands clasped, lift your arms and rock all the way to one side (Figure 7), then to the other. (Figure 8.) Rock back and forth, ten times to each side, in a continuous motion. This makes the back, shoulders, and hips flexible and thins the waistline.

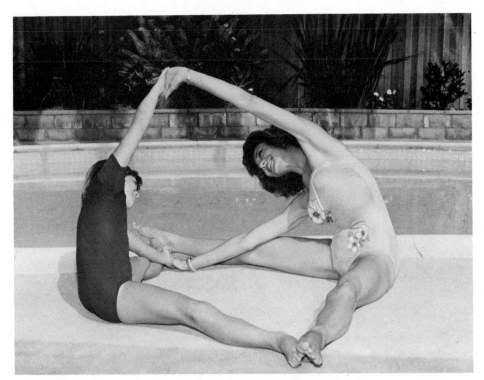

Figure 7.

Figure 8.

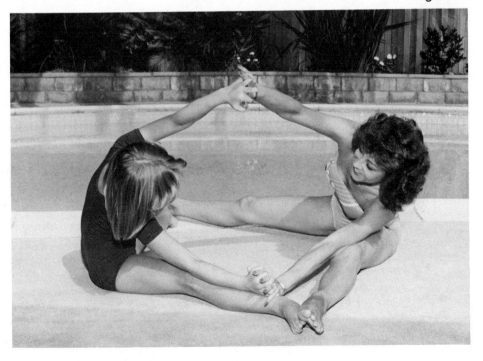

SOMETHING SPECIAL

Kids' Togetherness Rock

You have to teach your children to work together in exercise routines. Here I get Heather and Christy going with some TOGETHERNESS ROCK, moving back and forth and making marvelous music together. (Figures 9 and 10.)

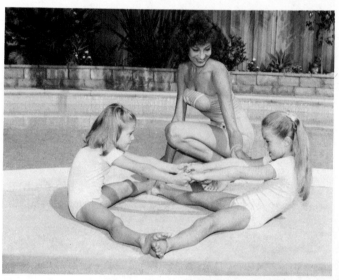

Figure 9.

Figure 10.

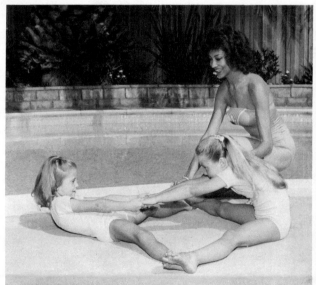

Kids' Togetherness Situps

It is difficult to devise effective three-way exercises, but there's always a way to keep the odd-one-out occupied. Here, my youngest helps by holding down the feet of her big sisters while they play sole-mates and do TO-GETHERNESS SITUPS. (Figures 11 and 12.)

Help your children grow up to be Beautiful People. Help your partner, and let him help you. Physical fitness isn't just for macho men nowadays; it's for everyone. Physical fitness is a family affair.

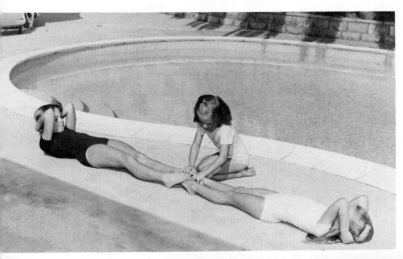

Figure 11.

Figure 12.

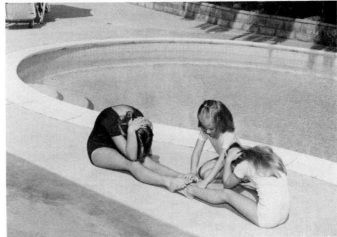

19
RELAXATION

THERE COMES A TIME when, in the words of Beverly Hills's most legendary landowner, Greta Garbo — who supposedly owns half of Rodeo Drive and other fancy streets hereabouts — "I vant to be alone." We all need some private time for ourselves. Exercise can provide relief from the tensions of the day, release from responsibilities, and relaxation that enables you to get your head on straight and your act together. (Pardon the show-biz jargon, but in Beverly Hills we're close to Hollywood!)

SOMETHING SPECIAL

The Cobra

Try a COBRA. Lie flat on your stomach, with your hands placed palms-down under your shoulders and your forehead touching the floor. (Figure 1.) Now, raise your upper body, pulling your head back and tightening your buttocks, and hold for a short time. (Figure 2.) Then, slowly lower yourself to the floor and relax with your arms at your sides. But don't fall asleep. Repeat the Cobra a few times. Afterwards, you should feel like warm syrup spreading over pancakes.

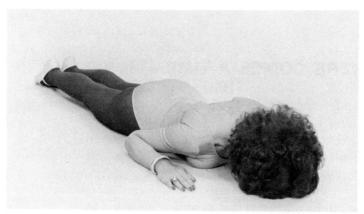

Figure 1.

Figure 2.

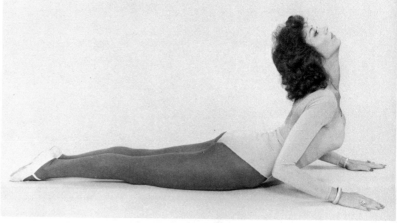

Head Rolls

Now do some HEAD ROLLS. Let your head roll in a circular motion forward (Figure 3), to the side, back (Figure 4), and to the other side, as if it were not attached to your body. Use a gentle rolling motion. Relax the rest of your body as much as possible. Feel the tension drift away.

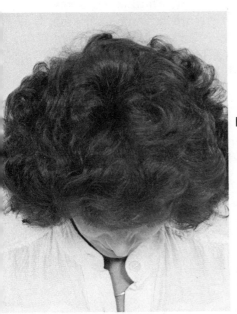

Figure 3.

Figure 4.

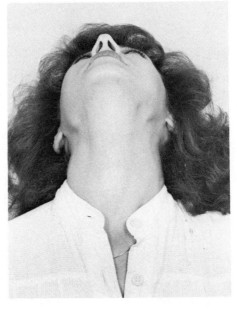

Yoga Sit

Finish with a YOGA SIT — any one of the variations. Here is one of the most relaxed. (Figure 5.) Clear your mind as completely as possible. Think of the color white. Or a blank wall. Concentrate on a word that will relax you, like "love," and say it slowly over and over again in your mind. If you prefer, think of a field of wildflowers, snow-capped mountains, a mountain stream, a home in Beverly Hills. . . .

Other relaxation exercises include the Horizontal Stretch in Chapter 1, Head Presses and Stretches in Chapter 3, the Hail Hero and Yoga Sit in Chapter 6, Rotation and Kneeling Stretches in Chapter 7, the Shoulder Shrugs and Rib Cage Raises in Chapter 11, and the Yoga Sits and Hail Heroes in Chapter 17. Stretch out for success. Gain your goals of good health and good looks. Be beautiful.

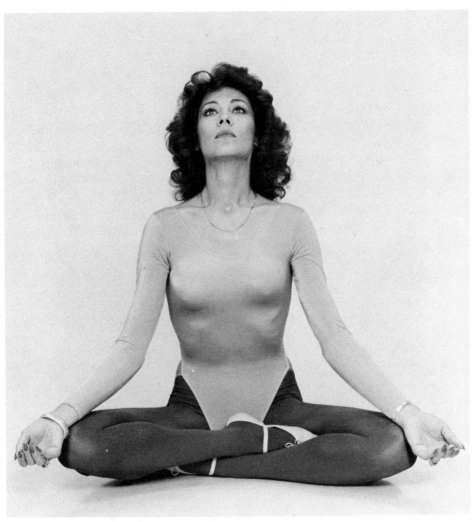

Figure 5.

20
SKIN CARE

EXERCISE DOES WONDERS for the outer you as well as the inner you. The sort of easy but effective exercises I have recommended not only will build you up and slim you down but will improve the blood circulation and the supply of oxygen throughout your body. This in turn will produce a naturally healthy skin coloring and complexion. The exercise not only will make your body more limber, but will restore elasticity in your skin.

Throughout these exercises I have encouraged deep breathing — inhaling through the nose, exhaling through the mouth. We all breathe, of course. But we do not all breathe correctly. We have to breathe deeply. And we have to seek out, at least periodically, areas where the air is not contaminated — not easy to find these days.

Proper breathing can be the greatest relaxer of all. Rhythmic, even breathing, especially in a Yoga Sit, for a few minutes before bedtime will relax your muscles for a good night's sleep. It also will relax your skin. And your mind. You do not have to meditate, though a relaxed mind produces a relaxed body.

Diet and the Skin

A good diet does wonders for you externally as well as internally. It is true to a great extent that you are what you eat. Your body and your physical conditioning reflect not only the exercise you get, but the food you eat. Carbohydrates and fats provide energy, but if you eat too much rich or starchy food, too much sweet or junk food, your body will soften, your fitness fade and your mental attitude deteriorate.

I am not going into detail about diet here, nor will I lecture you. I will remind you that tobacco smoke dilates the arteries, slows down the circulation of blood throughout your body and decreases the lungs' capacity; that cholesterol coats and narrows the arteries; and that alcohol works hardships on the liver and other organs and brings small blood vessels to the surface, where they materialize as spiderweb veins or splotches of red. It is as bad for your external skin as it is for your internal organs to smoke or drink, especially to excess, or to eat too many unhealthful foods.

It is no secret that it is important to eat a balanced diet of nutritious foods. You need protein in your diet as well as carbohydrates. You do not need a lot of sugar. It is preferable to get the essential nutrients from a good diet, but I feel that vitamins are good insurance becuase of the overprocessing of so much of today's food. Fresh fruits and vegetables supply the nutrients you need, as long as they are properly cooked — which means not overcooked. I have nothing against beef, but I do believe you should vary your diet with fish and fowl. Fry your food infrequently. Salads — without rich dressings — are great. Dairy foods are fine, but do not overdo them. The older you get, the less milk you need.

Water is the most underrated health drink. Coffee, tea, and soft drinks consist primarily of water, but they also bring into your system substances it doesn't need. Pure water does not. If your area does not have pure water, boil it, cool it off, and keep it cold in bottles in the refrigerator. Or buy good bottled water. But drink six to ten glasses a day. If you are fit, your body will use it well. Water flushes wastes out of your body. And nourishes and moisturizes the skin.

Testing Your Skin

To a certain extent, your skin reflects your physical condition. But sometimes it can contrast with your physical condition. A poor complexion can make you look unhealthy even if you are in good physical condition. Whether your skin is good or bad or something in between, there are things you can do to improve it and to keep it looking good.

Begin by determining what type of skin you have — dry or oily, stiff or elastic. If you don't want to take the trouble to get a professional skin analysis, there are less exact but adequate ways to judge for yourself.

Taking a good, close look at yourself is one. Get within three inches of a mirror, preferably a magnifying mirror, and study your skin. If the pores are enlarged and shiny, you are secreting oils. Usually, you will have been suffering from blackheads or other forms of acne. If the pores are tight and the skin is flaky, you have dry skin.

Pinch about three inches of skin between your thumb and forefinger. You can tell whether it is soft or hard. If it snaps back immediately when you release it, it still has elasticity. Usually, the elasticity of the skin starts to diminish in a person's early twenties. Excessive exposure to the sun accelerates this process. The less elastic the skin, the sooner wrinkles appear. Your usual facial expressions produce lines around the eyes and mouth. Your chin and neck start to sag. Now is the time to do something about it. It's even better if you can do something before the sagging and wrinkling begin, or before they get too advanced. The Funny Face facial exercises will help a lot. So will other things.

Problems

The most common reaction people have to skin problems is to overreact. If they have acne, they get the strongest remedy they can find to combat it, often a preparation that is highly alkaline and extremely drying. They dry up their oily areas, perhaps, but they dry up the rest of their skin too — to the point where it starts to flake off. Some medications that can be bought in drugstores and department stores are extremely strong. The skin is very delicate. While oily skin has to be corrected, to rob it of all its natural moisture will only cause other problems. Mild medications that attack problem areas with some restraint and do the job gradually and thoroughly without shocking the skin into other problems are preferable by far. A doctor's advice might be worthwhile here.

If your skin is allergic to specific things, from dust to flowers, and tends to become discolored or to swell or to develop rashes, you require a doctor's specific treatment. But perhaps you simply have sensitive skin. In either case, you probably should limit yourself to hypoallergenic soaps, skin-care products, and cosmetics. These are fragrance-free and contain fewer strong chemical irritants than other preparations. However, be aware that even they are not totally without the chemicals that may irritate your skin. Purchase these cosmetics more often and in smaller amounts than usual, because hypoallergenic products are made without preservatives. Check with a qualified person about the ingredients in a product before purchasing it.

Moisturizers

One of the best things you can do for your skin beyond exercising it is to moisturize it regularly. Not only those of you who have dry skin, but those who have oily skin, too. Many of the entertainers who frequent my salon have problem skin that has been dried out by the extremely hot lights under which they work and by the heavy stage and screen makeup they must use. They need moisturizers for their faces. They often need and want them on their necks and shoulders, too. Oily skin requires less moisturizing, but even oily skin usually needs it around the eyes, the mouth, and the throat.

Moisturizers may be the most misunderstood of beauty aids. They do not change the skin type. But while there is no metabolic change, most do soften the skin without penetrating it. Instead, moisturizers act to protect the skin against water loss which will lead to dryness and eventually can cause wrinkles. As a coating, moisturizers do slow down the secretion of body oils and perspiration, but the body needs to do some of this to keep its proper temperature and to maintain the regular replacement of skin cells.

Use refined products with a liquid or lanolin base rather than those with an oil base, no matter what the claims of "penetration" made by the manufacturers. Emollient creams are fine, since they act as softeners and protectors like the others; but thick humectants, which are like petroleum jellies, may make the skin seem soft, while actually they may be making the skin drier.

The more expensive moisturizers are not necessarily the more effective ones. Usually the added cost is for ingredients such as perfumes which add no protection. Apply a moisturizer immediately after washing or showering, when the skin contains the moisture you want to preserve. Apply it sparingly. A little dab will do you. Spread it thoroughly from above your breasts, up over your throat to your chin, and over your face. Include your ears and the back of your neck. Rather than using more, apply less more often. Moisturizers do not stay on forever, especially in the summer when you perspire more and wash your face more often. Your skin type will determine the amount and type of moisturizing you require. Naturally, if you are over twenty-five and have a dry, flaky skin, you should use a product which is concentrated while refined enough to penetrate the skin. You might use a lighter moisturizer during the day.

It should take less than half a minute to apply a moisturizer, and it is preferable to blot off any excess after about ten minutes. This "second skin" becomes the base for anything else you apply to your skin afterwards.

Toners

Everyone can use toners, from the mildest kinds made from herbal extracts to the strongest types of astringents for oily and acne skin. The more oily the skin, the stronger the toner it needs; the drier the skin, the milder the toner. There also are exfoliating products made with a granular substance that are very effective in dissolving the dead cells that accumulate on the surface of dry skin and restoring to the skin its natural blush and healthy look.

Your skin type will determine the type of toner you need and how often it should be used. Smooth it on gently, with a circular motion. It is best to use sterile cotton balls to apply it in upward strokes, starting from the neck. Avoid the fragile skin area around the eyes. A toner may be applied after cleansing the face and before a moisturizing base is put on.

Eye Creams

Specially formulated eye creams should be used to condition the area around the eyes. Of a heavier consistency than the normal moisturizers, they are less likely to leak into the eye itself. Apply these from the cheekbones up, and around the underside of the eye socket. Do not apply them above the eyes. It is the underside where a cream is needed most anyway, since this is where dry skin and wrinkles begin to form.

Masks

Skin masks and facial packs help in various ways to soothe, stimulate, tone, cleanse, and moisturize the skin. They take a little time, say twenty to thirty minutes, to do a proper job, so you would be wise to use them when you have ample time before going out for the evening, or before going to bed at night.

Incidentally, you can make up your own natural packs that are every bit as effective as the prepared products available in the stores. Actually, vitamins can be applied to the skin which will be absorbed by the skin, often in the form of fresh fruits and vegetables. It might be fun to experiment with these. One compound that is effective on mature skin which has lost elasticity and is starting to wrinkle consists of two tablespoons of yeast mixed with a few drops of distilled water and blended into a paste. This mixture stimulates the growth of new skin cells. If your skin is especially dry, you might add two drops of Vitamin E to the mixture to lubricate the skin. Another suggestion that works well for dry skin is to blend a banana, using part of its skin, with a tablespoon of honey to form a moisturizing pack. Also, a blend of peaches and honey is effective. Use a blender for preparing your natural beauty aids. Apply them all over the face, being careful around the eyes.

An application of grated raw potato will lighten dark areas around the eyes and reduce puffiness. Grated cucumbers also work well around the eyes. And a slice of cucumber laid on the eyelids will soothe the eyes. For an oily skin, grind grapefruit to a fine pulp, skin and all, and apply to the face to slow down the excess secretion of oils. Or use a liquefied tomato or a liquefied, cored apple. For excessively oily skin, add a tablespoon of lemon juice to each of these preparations. Outlandish though some of these concoctions may seem, the skin will absorb and put to good use the natural vitamins they provide. The more natural the source of the vitamins, the more effective the preparations.

Gels made from herbal, plant, and flower extracts are extremely effective in temporarily restoring the natural moisture of the skin and erasing the fine lines that develop at day's end.

Also available these days are gels made from the cactus-type aloe vera plant, which many consider a miracle medicine. I do not believe in miracles, but I am amazed at how quickly this gel heals cuts, bruises, scrapes, and so forth. I do not know if it will work all the wonders claimed for it, but I do recommend it as a mask to help heal sore or sensitive skin. Apply it sparingly, though, as it is extremely expensive.

When you go to bed, do not plan to leave your mask on overnight. All masks should be removed and the skin rinsed and cleansed thoroughly after twenty to thirty minutes.

220

Beyond the Face

Moisturizers, toners, and even some masks should be applied not only to the face, ears, and neck, but also the shoulders, arms, hands, legs, and feet at times, depending on the problem. There are specific products for specific parts of the body. You have done only half the job if you have taken care of your face and not your neck, upper chest, or shoulders. You certainly haven't done the job if you haven't taken care of your hands.

Exfoliating creams of a granular consistency or pumice stones slicked with soap are recommended for the removal of the dry skin that forms on your elbows, knees, and heels. For removing hair from underarms and legs there are three methods: shaving with a safety razor, body waxing, and dipilatories. Depilatories can be irritating so use them with caution.

Cleansing

The very best thing you can do for your skin is to keep it clean. Wash frequently and thoroughly. Wash your hands and face carefully before applying anything to your face. Avoid alkaline soaps or harsh detergents and highly perfumed soaps, especially for the face. Use mild soaps with a lanolin base or natural biogenic soaps made from herbal or plant extracts, and use water-soluble cleansers on the face whenever possible.

Keep your skin clean and you will be helping to keep it healthy. Keep your skin clean and you will feel good and smell good. Use perfumes sparingly to enhance your natural scents. Never use them so heavily that they become you and are the first and often the only thing others notice about you.

Be sure your skin is completely clean before you apply anything to it, and rinse off thoroughly anything you apply to your skin after it has had its chance to do something for you. This is especially true of makeup, which tends to become embedded in the pores and should be thoroughly removed before retiring.

Makeup

Use daytime makeup sparingly and wisely to maximize your assets and minimize your liabilities. Use good, fresh makeup. The most expensive brands are not necessarily the best, but the least expensive ones are often the worst. I don't want to touch on specific brands here, but experiment until you find the ones that work best for you and your skin.

Always apply makeup over clean skin that is protected by a moisturizer. Apply it in natural lighting or whatever is similar to what exists in your world. Use lighter, brighter makeup for outdoor and daytime activities, and heavier, more dramatic makeup for indoor and nighttime activities. I know one actress who is wise enough to insist that her makeup be applied on the set, with the lighting that will be used in each scene, rather than in a differently lit makeup room out back somewhere. Never judge makeup by a dab on the back of the hand, but by a short stroke on the area on which it is to be used, such as a cheekbone.

Apply all makeup over a light foundation that matches your own skin tone, usually one with a liquid base. Apply the foundation with your fingertips and blend with a clean sponge. Foundation creams come in oil or oil-free bases. If you have problems with acne or blemishes, try an oil-free makeup. Talk to a qualified person about your skin type before selecting a foundation.

Use specially formulated sticks or creams under the

eyes or on dark spots, acne, or other blemishes. Do not use more or heavier makeup simply because you have deep wrinkles, because the makeup will tend to collect in the wrinkles and emphasize them rather than cover them. Since liquids and creams tend to become embedded in creases, use a powder or a pencil in these areas.

Always apply makeup from the inside of the face and work outward. Begin at the forehead and chin, then go to the cheeks. Lightly brush fine facial hairs downward for a finished look. Use translucent powders which reflect normal skin tones. Remember that it is more difficult to keep a uniform look with creams than with powders. Creams do tend to give a soft, dewy look, but powders are easier to apply in the exact amounts desired.

Do not overdo it. Work with the natural color of your skin and the skeletal structure of your face to emphasize those areas that are most attractive and deemphasize those that are the least attractive. Use less, and more conservative, makeup for everyday; more, and brighter, makeup for evenings out. But unless you are out to shock, do not use so much that it is the makeup others notice, not your face.

The eyes and mouth are the two most important features, and special care should be taken to apply makeup to them for the most pleasing effect. Using a lighter shade of coloring on your lips will make your eyes seem larger. If you want a dewy look for your lips, use a lip gloss, but remember that it will not last as long as a cream. Use a lip pencil to outline your lips first, then fill in the inside with up-and-down strokes rather than side-to-side strokes for the best effect. Pencils or fine brushes are best for applying eye shadow and eye liner and to touch up the eyebrows properly. It pays to invest in professional-quality equipment for applying makeup.

Some women do not use makeup wisely and would be better off without it. In any event you should remove it carefully and completely at the end of the day, or sooner if you dare. Do not use a washcloth with soap and water to scrub off makeup, especially around the eyes. Instead, use soft, clean cotton pads treated with makeup remover, and change them frequently as you remove the day's grime. Make upward strokes, except around the eyes, where you should stroke from the inside out and around the eye in a circular motion. After removing makeup, wash your face and other areas that were made up. Cleanse your skin completely. Always use cool or lukewarm water; never use hot or cold, which shocks the skin. Use gentle soaps on your face. Pat dry. Apply the protection of a moisturizer.

Exercise

We are back to exercise. Through exercising you will achieve the fitness you want and the skin condition that will make you as attractive as you possibly can be. Exercise promotes the circulation of blood and oxygen throughout your body that gives your skin a healthy glow, softness, and elasticity. Once again, whether you live in Beverly Hills or wherever, you can be one of the Beautiful People.